MOVE
CHILL

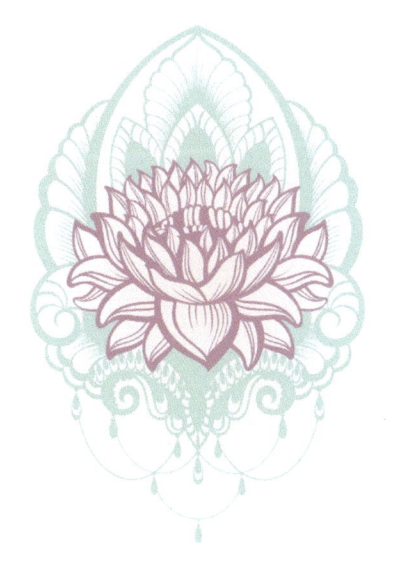

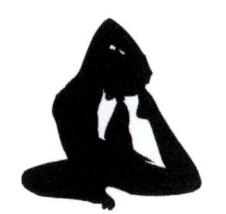

YOGA

YOGA CLASS PLANS, VOLUME 1

12 adaptable class plans for yoga teachers

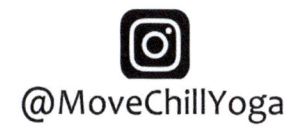

@MoveChillYoga

Rita Rainieri Polak

Copyright © 2018 by Rita Rainieri-Polak. All rights reserved.

This book may not be reproduced in whole or in part without written permission from the publisher. Nor may any part of this book be reproduced, stored in a retrieval system, or transmitted in any form or by any means, electronic, mechanical, photocopying, recording, or other, without written permission from the publisher.

ISBN-13:
978-1984014573

ISBN-10:
1984014579

VOLUME I

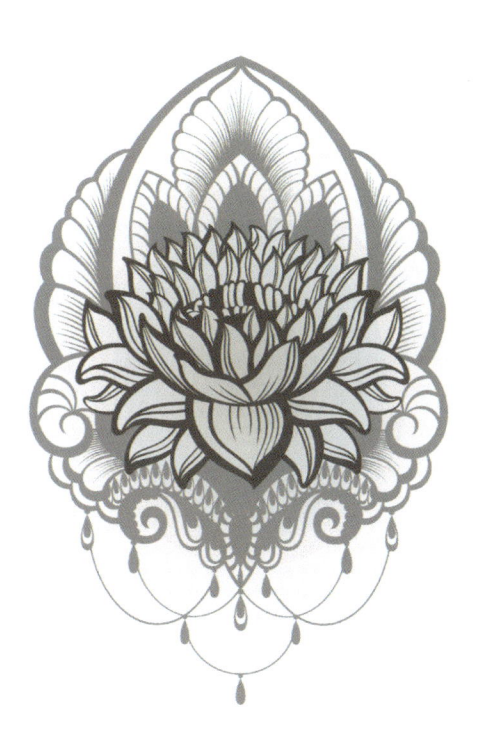

Table of Contents

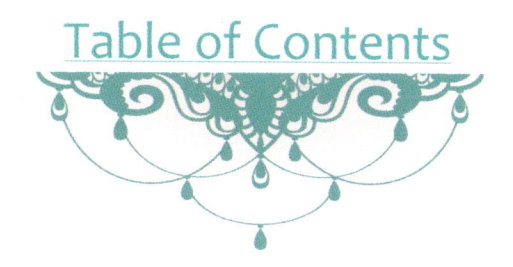

Disclaimer

INTRODUCTION

MOVE CHILL TEACH

YOGA CLASS PLAN 1 - **HAPPINESS BOOST**

YOGA CLASS PLAN 2 - **JOURNEY**

YOGA CLASS PLAN 3 – **COLOR THE MIND**

YOGA CLASS PLAN 4 – **LIVING IN THE MOMENT**

YOGA CLASS PLAN 5 – **POWER WITHIN**

YOGA CLASS PLAN 6 – **BREATH IS LIFE**

YOGA CLASS PLAN 7 – **A PRACTICE FOR COLDER SEASONS**

YOGA CLASS PLAN 8 – **A PRACTICE FOR WARMER SEASONS**

YOGA CLASS PLAN 9 - **TRADITIONAL**

YOGA CLASS PLAN 10 - **GRATITUDE**

YOGA CLASS PLAN 11 – **LETTING GO**

YOGA CLASS PLAN 12 – **STRENGTH & BALANCE**

PLAYLISTS

NOTES

Disclaimer

This book is for informational purposes only and is meant to enhance but not replace professional medical care, medical advice, or exercise.
All forms of movement pose some inherent risk.
The author advises readers to take full responsibility for their safety and the safety of students.
As with all exercise programs, proper discretion should be top of mind. Consult a healthcare professional before participating in the techniques described within this book's collection.

INTRODUCTION

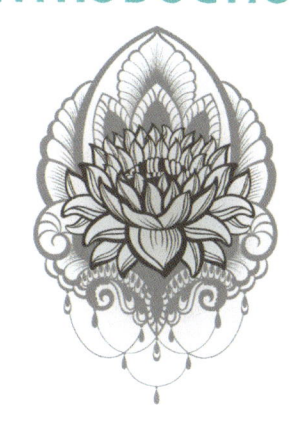

Whether you're just starting to teach yoga, or you have years of yoga teaching experience, you will likely develop a desire or need to infuse fresh ideas and dynamic sequences into your yoga classes and everyday practice. This book is meant to partner with you in that effort, and will be a welcome addition to your everyday practice and yoga class planning.

Planning beneficial and enjoyable yoga classes can be time consuming and sometimes challenging in today's busy lifestyle.
As a yoga teacher with a full schedule, it's an essential luxury to experience a class that another yoga teacher has thoughtfully planned. For yoga teachers who are just starting to teach, it can be extremely useful to find accessible and succinct class plans that can assist in developing your own style and furthering your practice.

When the planning endeavor is completed and laid out for you, the added benefits of reduced stress will allow you to present more of your energy to your students and will benefit the spirit of your classes.

Most importantly, you can use these class plans to serve as a framework in creating your own. Enjoy implementing your personal variations, flows, and transitions to make them yours.

Namaste

Rita
@MoveChillYoga

MOVE CHILL TEACH

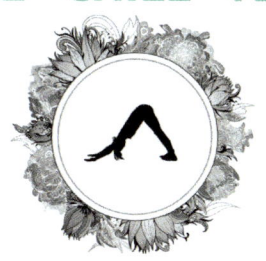

Explore
Twelve 40-60 minute classes

All classes include variations on the following:
Opening: Meditation or grounding
Movement: Asanas and Flows
Closing: Savasana + Meditation/Yoga Nidra

Each class plan is outlined with 2 tools:

A) YOGA CLASS PLAN
This presents the written illustration of the class from opening to closing; Includes meditations, physical practice, alignment cues, Sanskrit posture names and pronunciations, and guided imagery.

B) PORTABLE QUICK REFERENCE
Portable notes designed for practice. This is a perfect practice tool for ease of memorization.

* You can also tuck this sheet under the corner of your mat or next to your mat for quick reference as you practice to teach your class.

TIPS FOR THE NEW YOGA TEACHER
- Holding the postures for 4-5 breath counts is recommended.
- While experiencing the sequences, you'll sense where you'd like to focus, edit, add, or linger a bit longer. Examples: You may want to lengthen or shorten meditations where appropriate, incorporate chanting, implement hands-on adjustments, or add/edit more advanced postures.
- Throughout the practice, it is important to allow for pauses and natural space.
- Gently guide your students to breathe during these pauses and all through the practice.

1
happiness boost

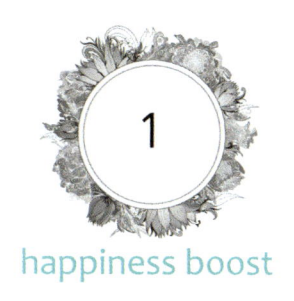

Opening Meditation
bliss & well-being

Sit in Easy Pose Sukhasana (Soo- KAHS-uh-nah)
Close your eyes, face palms up to bring in energy.

Get comfortable. Draw your attention to your breath.

Recall the feeling of happiness and what that means to you.

On your next inhale, breathe in the feeling happiness and a sense of well-being. As you exhale, let go of any tension.

Let the warmth of happiness flow through your whole body, from the crown of your head all the way down to your toes.

Find your way to the full emotion of happiness and absorb the light and joy it delivers. Feel your body relaxed and your mind peaceful and open.

Imagine or dream up a time and place where you are experiencing bliss and happiness. Or, recall a time when you experienced the fullness of happiness, laughter, and well-being. With family or good friends? A safe and special place?

Bring the image of the moment to mind.

Dive into how the experience of happiness and well-being feels in your body. Take a few moments to feel the sensations in your body and that mood in your mind.

Relax into it more with each inhale and exhale.

Continuing the gentle **breathing flow** with **shoulder rolls**:
Sitting up tall lengthening from the crown of head.
Inhale lift shoulders high
Exhale roll shoulders back and down
Inhale lift shoulders high
Exhale roll shoulders back and down
Repeat X 3

Both arms all the way up inhale
Exhale the arms down
X 3

Side body stretch
Lift the left arm up and overhead, placing the right hand on the mat at your side
Reach over, stretching the side body. Breathe into the stretch
Both arms up to Center
Repeat, lifting and stretching the right arm over

Seated spinal twist Parivrtta Sukhasana variation (pah-ruh-VREE-tah soo-KAHS-uh-nah)
Place right hand on floor behind. Bring left hand to outside of right knee, twisting to the right.
Exhale gently, gazing over the right shoulder
Breathe into the twist
Come back to center – arms up
Repeat on other side twisting the other way

Align yourself to be in the present moment. One thing at a time

Table Pose Bharmanasana (Bar-man-AHS-un-nah)
Place arms directly under shoulders, extend the neck and allow the back to be flat.
Press the tail bone towards the back wall and the crown of the head towards the front wall, lengthening the spine.
Warming up spine, move into **Cat Pose** Marjaryasana (Mahr-jahr-ee-AHS-uh-nah)
Inhale tuck tailbone, round the back, head strait, then down
Cow Pose Bitilasana (Bi-til-AHS-uh-nah)
Exhale arch your back, pushing shoulders back, head comes up
Repeat Cat/Cow X3
Go at your own pace, 2 or more deep breaths

Tuck the toes and push back to
Downward Dog Adho Mukha Svanasana (AH-doh MOO-kah-shvah-Nahs-ana)
Deep breath - All 10 fingers and palms pressing into mat, hips lifting up as if a string is pulling up the hips, gaze at the belly button
Find stillness

Walk up to **Standing Forward Bend** Uttanasana (OO-tan-AHS-un-nah)
Keep a flat back coming up to **Mountain Pose** Tadasana (Ta-DAHS-un-nah)
Stand strong, bring hands together at heart center. Recall again the sensation of happiness from the opening meditation. Pause and fix the mind here for 3 breath cycles.

Arms up and over head inhale, Exhale dive forward keeping the back flat
Forward bend Uttanasana all the way down again stretching a bit deeper this time
Roll back up to **Mountain Pose** Tadasana
Exhale **Forward bend** Uttanasana all the way down once more
Jump or walk back to **Plank Pose** Kumbhakasana (koom-bahk-AHS-uh-nuh)
Hold for 1 breath cycle
Knees chest chin come down **Cobra** Bhujangasana (boo-jang-GAHS-uh-nah)
Hug elbows in, Press down through tops of feet. Inhale gently lift head and chest, shoulders back, heart forward. Gaze to the floor or up to the sky.

Tuck toes under for **Down Dog Split RIGHT LEG** Tri Pada Adho Mukha Svanasana (Tri Pada AH-doh MOO-kah-shvah-Nahs-ana)
RIGHT leg lifts. Hips level and square with the floor, hold for 1 breath
Hug and squeeze right knee in and bring right leg forward between hands
Lift into **Warrior I** Virabhadrasana I (Veer-ah-bah-DRAHS-ana)
Right foot out 90 degrees, front thigh parallel to floor, Back foot flat and toes turned out slightly. Shoulders over hips, arms reaching up, heart is open and light.
Outstretch arms into **Warrior II** Virabhadrasana II
Relax shoulders down. INHALE. Wide stance with heel to heel alignment.
Straiten front leg and EXHALE.
Bend leg back to **Warrior II** and INHALE
Straiten front leg and EXHALE
Bend leg back to **Warrior II** and INHALE
Straiten front leg and EXHALE

Cartwheel arms and hands down to frame the front foot
Both feet back to **Plank Pose** Kumbhakasana
Hold for 1 breath cycle
Knees chest chin come down **Cobra** Bhujangasana
Hug elbows in, Press down through tops of feet. Inhale gently lift head and chest, shoulders back, heart forward. Gaze to the floor or up to the sky.
Pause for 1 breath cycle

Tuck toes under for **Down Dog Split LEFT LEG** Tri Pada Adho Mukha Svanasana
LEFT leg lifts. Hips level and square with the floor, hold for 1 breath
Hug and squeeze left knee in and bring the left leg forward between hands
Lift into **Warrior I** Virabhadrasana I (Veer-ah-bah-DRAHS-ana)
Left foot out 90 degrees, front thigh parallel to floor, back foot flat and toes turned out slightly. Shoulders over hips, arms reaching up, heart is open and light.
Outstretch arms into **Warrior II** Virabhadrasana II
Relax shoulders down. INHALE. Wide stance with heel to heel alignment.
Straiten front leg and EXHALE.
Bend leg back to **Warrior II** and INHALE
Straiten front leg and EXHALE
Bend leg back to **Warrior II** and INHALE
Straiten front leg and EXHALE

Cartwheel arms and hands down to frame the front foot
Both feet back to **Plank Pose** Kumbhakasana

Hold for 1 breath cycle
Knees chest chin come down **Cobra** Bhujangasana
Hug elbows in, Press down through tops of feet. Inhale gently lift head and chest, shoulders back, heart forward. Gaze to the floor or up to the sky.
Pause for 1 breath cycle
Lift to **Upward Dog** Urdhva Mukha Svanasana (OORD-vah MOO-kah shvon-AHS-anna)
Straitening arms. Keep shoulders relaxed. Hold for 3 breaths

Move to **Table** Bharmanasana
Lift the RIGHT arm all the way up skyward twisting the front body, look at top hand
Breathe and hold for 2 counts of breath
Eye of the needle Sucirandhrasana (Sucir-ahn-Dhrah-suh-nah)
Scoop the right arm down under the front body, resting right shoulder on the floor, arm outstretched flat on the mat, palm now facing up.
Back to center **Table** Bharmanasana
Switch sides, Lifting LEFT arm skyward twisting front body, look at top hand
Breathe and hold for 2 counts of breath
Eye of the needle Sucirandhrasana with LEFT arm
Scoop the left arm down under front body, resting left shoulder on the floor, arm outstretched flat on the mat, palm now facing up.

Tuck toes **Down Dog Split RIGHT LEG** Tri Pada Adho Mukha Svanasana
RIGHT leg lifts Hips level and square with the floor, hold for 1 breath
Hug and squeeze right knee in and bring right leg forward between hands
Warrior I Virabhadrasana I
Right foot out in front, leg at 90 degrees, front thigh parallel to floor, Back foot flat and toes turned out slightly. Shoulders over hips, arms reaching up, heart is open and light.
Warrior III Virabhadrasana III
Keep both hips level and pointing toward the floor as you fully extend your left leg back. Flex the left foot and keep the toes pointing down at the floor. Actively engage the muscles of the right leg. Bring your arms back along your sides. Pause and balance, finding an un-moving point of focus or **drishti** for balance. Breathe.
Step to **Mountain Pose** Tadasana
Move into **1-legged Chair Pose** Eka Pada Utkatasana (Eeka-pah-duh Oot-Kah –TAS –uh-nah)
Hugging in the right leg. Bend your left knee as if sitting.
Pause. Now straiten left leg.
Extend your right leg out in front, grabbing the outer edge side of the right foot with your left hand for **Revolved Hand to big toe** Parivrtta Hasta Padangusthasana
(Pari Vri-TUH HAHS-tuh pahd-ahng-goosh-TAHS-uh-nuh)
Twist from the waist to the right side of the space, and extend your right arm out behind. Balance. Breathe. Hug your right leg back in.
Bend your left leg, and step the right leg back to **Warrior I** Virabhadrasana I
Cartwheel arms down to frame the front foot
Jump or walk back to **Plank Pose** Kumbhakasana
Hold for 1 breath cycle
Knees chest chin come down **Cobra** Bhujangasana
Hug elbows in, Press down through tops of feet. Inhale gently lift head and chest, shoulders back, heart forward. Gaze to the floor or up to the sky.

Pause for 1 breath cycle

Down Dog Split LEFT LEG Tri Pada Adho Mukha Svanasana
LEFT leg lifts Hips level and square with the floor, hold for 1 breath
Hug and squeeze left knee in and bring left leg forward between hands
Warrior I Virabhadrasana I
Left foot out in front, leg at 90 degrees, front thigh parallel to floor, Back foot flat and toes turned out slightly. Shoulders over hips, arms reaching up, heart is open and light.
Warrior III Virabhadrasana III
Keep both hips level and pointing toward the floor as you fully extend your right leg back. Flex the right foot and keep the toes pointing down at the floor. Actively engage the muscles of the left leg. Bring your arms back along your sides. Pause and balance, finding an un-moving point of focus or **drishti** for balance. Breathe.
Step to **Mountain Pose** Tadasana
Move into **1-legged Chair Pose** Eka Pada Utkatasana (Eeka-pah-duh Oot-Kah –TAS –uh-nah)
Hugging in the left leg. Bend your right knee as if sitting.
Pause. Now straiten right leg.
Extend your left leg out in front, grabbing the outer edge side of the left foot with your right hand for **Revolved Hand to big toe** Parivrtta Hasta Padangusthasana
(Pari Vri-TUH HAHS-tuh pahd-ahng-goosh-TAHS-uh-nuh)
Twist from the waist to the left side of the space, and extend your left arm out behind. Balance. Breathe. Hug your left leg back in.
Bend your right leg, and step the left leg back to **Warrior I** Virabhadrasana I

Cartwheel arms down to frame the front foot
Jump or walk back to **Plank Pose** Kumbhakasana
Hold for 1 breath cycle
Knees chest chin come down **Cobra** Bhujangasana
Hug elbows in, Press down through tops of feet. Inhale gently lift head and chest, shoulders back, heart forward. Gaze to the floor or up to the sky.
Pause for 1 breath cycle

Balancing Table Dandayamna Bharmanasana variation
(Dan-day-AHM-nuh Bar-man-AHS-ah-nuh)
From Table, Lift RIGHT leg, extend LEFT arm
Bend RIGHT leg skyward. Swim left arm around and reach back to grab the top of your right foot into **Lord of the Dance variation** Natarajasana (not-ah-raj-AHS-uh-nah)
Lift and extend the leg up as you hold
Push back to **Child's Pose** Balasana (bah-LAHS-ah-nuh)
Extend arms out, melt heart down, place forehead to mat, knees apart
Pause for 5 breaths

Balancing Table Dandayamna Bharmanasana variation
(Dan-day-AHM-nuh Bar-man-AHS-ah-nuh)
From Table, Lift LEFT leg, extend RIGHT arm
Bend LEFT leg skyward. Swim right arm around and reach back to grab the top of your left foot into **Lord of the Dance variation** Natarajasana (not-ah-raj-AHS-uh-nah)
Lift and extend the leg up as you hold

Back to **Child's Pose** Balasana
Extend arms out, melt heart down, place forehead to mat, knees apart
Pause for 3-5 breaths.

Move onto the back and hug knees into chest for
Rock & Roll Jhulana Ludhakana variation (Jul-AHN-nuh Lood-HAK-ah-nuh)
Knees tucked, chin tucked, round the spine and gently roll back and then roll to sit up.
Repeat x 3

Bring your awareness again to the sensation of happiness from the opening meditation.
Pause and fix the mind here for 3 breath cycles.

Bridge flow:
Lay back down on the mat with the soles of the feet on the mat, knees up
Bridge Pose Setu Bahdha Sarvangasana (SAY-too-BAHN-duh Shar-vahn-GAHS-ah-nuh)
Windshied wiper the legs back and forth a few times, Draw your attention inward
Deep breath of happiness for taking this time out for you.
Walk heels up slightly toward sit bones
Arms down spread palms wide on mat. Slowly lift hip points up.
INHALE Open palms up skyward now as you lift the whole center body
EXHALE release down
INHALE lift hip points skyward
EXHALE release down
Repeating flow

Laying Body Twist Natrajasana (nah-traj-AHS-an-nuh)
Hug knees into chest and rock a little side to side.
Swing knees to the RIGHT and stack both knees on the ground to your RIGHT.
Arms out to a T.
Shoulder blades staying on the mat as much as possible while body is twisted. With each exhalation relax deeper into the pose.
Slowly turn head back to center. Hug knees into chest.
Swing knees to the LEFT and stack both knees on the ground to your LEFT.
Arms out to a T.
Shoulder blades staying on the mat as much as possible while body is twisted.
With each exhalation relax deeper into the pose. Slowly turn head back to center.
Hug knees into chest.

Inversion: **Candle Pose/Shoulderstand** Sarvangasana (sar-vang-AHS-uh-nah)
Inhale deeply while raising legs and spine until toes point skyward.
Place hands on center of spine between the waist and ribs to help lift up.
Body is resting on the shoulders and upper back, while your center is held up and supported with the hands.
Light your candle by flooding your mind with the sensation of happiness.
Hold for 3 counts of breath.
Bend knees and roll the hips and legs down gently.

Extend legs and arms and lay flat for **Relaxation Pose** Savasana (sha-VAHS-ah-nuh)
Allow the legs and feet to flop to the sides a little. Eyes are closed and relaxed.

Closing Meditation
holding happiness

Continue laying in **Relaxation pose** Savasana, or sit up into **Easy Pose** Sukasana

Count the breath to 10: Inhale deeply. PAUSE.
Then exhale, and at the very end of your out-breath, mentally count, "One."
Again, Inhale. PAUSE.
Exhale, and then at the end of your out-breath mentally count, "Two."

Keep counting like this at the end of every exhalation until "Ten".

For 1 week, continue to recall the sensation of happiness and well-being. You will find you can hold onto the feeling longer and longer.

If you are laying down, come up to a seat.
Bring your hands together at heart center. Namaste.

Move Chill Yoga
Portable Yoga Class Plan 1
happiness boost

tuck these portable plans beneath your mat for practice and/or reference

Breathing flow/shoulder roll
Side body stretch
Seated spinal twist
Table /Cat/Cow
Downward Dog
Standing Forward Bend
Mountain Pose
Recall the sensation of happiness and fix the mind here
Forward bend
Mountain Pose
Forward bend all the way down
Plank Pose
Cobra Pose

Down Dog Split RIGHT leg	**Down Dog Split LEFT leg**
Warrior I	**Warrior I**
Warrior II Straiten/Bend flow with breath	**Warrior II** Straiten/Bend flow with breath
Plank Pose	**Plank Pose**
Cobra Pose	**Cobra Pose**

Upward Dog
Table to Eye of the needle LEFT & RIGHT

Down Dog Split RIGHT leg	**Down Dog Split LEFT leg**
Warrior I	**Warrior I**
Warrior III	**Warrior III**
Mountain Pose	**Mountain Pose**
1-Leg Chair	**1-Leg Chair**
Revolved Hand to Big Toe	**Revolved Hand to Big Toe**
Warrior I	**Warrior I**
Plank Pose	**Plank Pose**
Cobra Pose	**Cobra Pose**

Balancing Table lift RIGHT leg	**Balancing Table** lift LEFT leg
Lord of the Dance variation	**Lord of the Dance variation**
Child's Pose	**Child's Pose**

Rock & Roll
Pause and recall the sensation of happiness
Bridge Flow
Laying Body Twist RIGHT & LEFT
Candle Pose/Shoulderstand
Flood the mind with the sensation of happiness
Relaxation Pose

2
journey

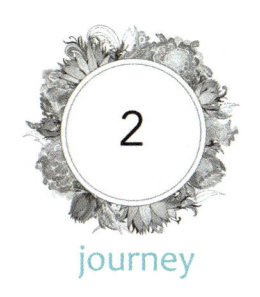

Opening Meditation
appreciating the journey of the breath

Sit in **Easy Pose** Sukhasana (Soo- KAHS-uh-nah), palms facing down to feel grounded.

Sit up tall as if you were being pulled skyward from the crown of your head.
Soften your mind. Soften your face. Soften the sides of the rib cage as well as the front abdominal wall. This will allow the breath to flow deeply and effectively.

In your mind, let your thoughts come up, and then come and go. Just observe them without giving them energy.
Instead, apply your awareness on the touch of the breath in the nostrils.
Feel the cool air come in like a soft deliberate breeze. Observe it fill deeply in the belly and up through the chest. On each inhale feel the breath expand. On the next inhale feel the breath now expand even further to fill into the sides of the ribcage.

Allow the breath to open and fill you will energy and calm.
In practicing this, your experience of breath awareness will strengthen.
Your breath will become deeply relaxing, and you will observe changes in the state of your consciousness.

The breath and these subtle changes are valuable companions to your yoga practice, but also impact and improve how we move through life.

Move to **Staff Pose** Dandasana (dan-DAHS-ah-nah)
Seated Twist with legs extended Parivrtta Sukhasana variation
(pah-ruh-VREE-tah soo-KAHS-uh-nah)
Cross right leg over left leg and bring right heel to outside of left knee. Inhale left hand to right knee, twisting to the RIGHT side space and exhale
Switch sides. Cross left leg over right leg and bring left heel to outside of right knee. Inhale right hand to left knee, twisting to the LEFT side space and exhale
Repeat both sides x 2

Still in **Staff Pose** Dandasana
Arms behind you fingers pointing towards body
Sit up tall, lifting arms up. Bend and fold forward from waist with a flat back
Inhale arms up, exhale bend from waist with a flat back
Grab toes or nearest point with hands and release your body, sink in and breathe.
Repeat x 3

Come up to sit into **Diamond Pose/Hero Pose** Vajrasana (vah-JRAHS-ah-nuh)
Sitting back on your heels, arms behind you, clasp hands and interlace fingers for
Rabbit Pose Sasangasana variation (sah-sang-AHS-uh-nuh)
Fold forward rolling onto the crown of head, lifting up clasped hands behind the body, and squeezing shoulder blades together.
Repeat Rabbit x 3

Sun Salutation A Surya Namaskara
With Sun Salutation A, practice breathing through the nose, which warms the air, just as the **vinyasa** warms up the body. Vin-YAHS-ah - **movement/flowing sequence in coordination with the breath**. Exhale when bending or folding and inhale when extending.

- Mountain pose Tadasana (Ta-DAHS-un-nah)
- Upward salute Urdhva Hastasana (Oord-vah hahs-TAHS-anna)
- Standing forward fold Uttanasana (Oo-tan-AHS-un-nah)
- Half forward fold Ardha Uttanasana (Ar-duh OO-tan-AHS-un-nah)
- High plank pose Utthita Chaturanga Dandasana into four-limbed staff pose Chaturanga Dandasana (oo-tee-tah chah-tuur-ANGH-uh dahn-DAHS-uh-nuh)
- Upward-facing dog Urdhva Mukha Svanasana (oord-vuh-Mookuh shvan-AHS-uh-na)
- Downward-facing dog Adho Mukha Svanasana (ahdo mookuh shvan-AHS-uh-na)
- Half forward fold Ardha Uttanasana
- Standing forward fold Uttanasana
- Upward salute Urdhva hastasana
- Mountain pose Tadasana

Repeat X 3

Move to **Table Pose** Bharmanasana (bar-ma-NAHS-ah-nah)
Tuck toes and push back to **Downward Dog** Adho Mukha Svanasana
(AH-doh MOO-kah-shvah-Nahs-ana)
Deep breath - All 10 fingers and palms pressing into mat, hips up as if a string is pulling up the hips skyward, gaze at belly button
Walk the dog bending 1 leg at a time. Neck and head are relaxed. Breathe.

Walk your feet further away. **Plank Pose** Kumbhakasana (koom-bahk-AHS-uh-nuh)
Reach crown of head forward - Inhale
Exhale into **Downward Dog** Adho Mukha Svanasana
Inhale **Plank Pose** Kumbhakasana
Alternating Dog & Plank x 3

Walk your feet between your hands
Inhale come all the way up **Mountain Pose** Tadasana
Stretch arms up and reach back
Exhale and fold down with a flat back into **Standing Forward Bend** Uttanasana
Alternate Mountain & Fold X 3

Stay in **Mountain Pose** Tadasana breathing arms up and down x 3
Now keeping arms up, Interlace fingers for **Standing Side Bend** Urdhva Hastasana (URD-vah Hast-AHS-uh-nuh) to the LEFT
Standing Side Bend Urdhva Hastasana to the RIGHT
Arms down. Come to top of mat.
Repeat x 3

Open your RIGHT leg back, toe pointing almost forward, left leg strait facing front.
Triangle Pose Utthita Trikonasana (oo-TEE-tah tree-koh-NAH-suh-nuh)
Inhale arms up and tip like a teapot, chest open, left arm to left foot.
*You can place a block behind your left foot and place hand here for stability.
Gaze upward, right arm is pointing up. Breathe.
Inhale come up keeping arms extend arms outward
Pushing through feet and hands, gaze forward, relax shoulders head and neck.
Repeat **Triangle Pose** Utthita Trikonasana X 2
On your next exhale, Bend the front leg to a 90 degree angle. Lean LEFT elbow to left thigh. Extend right arm up and gaze upward **Supported Side Stretch** Parsvakonasana (parsh-wah-cone-AHS-anna)
With left foot planted firmly into mat, raise RIGHT leg into **Tree pose** Vrksasana (vrik-SHAH-suh-nuh) arms up and out,
find a **drishti** point to focus your gaze and help with balance.

Back to **Mountain Pose** Tadasana at top of mat.
Open your LEFT leg back, toe pointing almost forward, right leg strait facing front.
Triangle Pose Utthita Trikonasana
Inhale arms up and tip like a teapot, chest open, right arm to right foot.

*You can place a block behind your right foot and place hand here for stability.
Gaze upward, left arm is pointing up. Breathe.
Inhale come up keeping arms extend arms outward
Pushing through feet and hands, gaze forward, relax shoulders head and neck.
Repeat **Triangle Pose** Utthita Trikonasana x 2
On your next exhale, Bend the front leg to a 90 degree angle. Lean RIGHT elbow to right thigh. Extend left arm up and gaze upward **Supported Side Stretch** Parsvakonasana
With right foot planted firmly into mat, raise LEFT leg into **Tree pose**
Vrksasana arms up and out, find an un-moving or **drishti** point to focus your gaze and help with balance.

Option: Have students stand in a circle to create a **Forest.** Everyone standing palm of hand to palm of hand, lifting hands and arms upward in **Tree pose** Vrksasana

From **Mountain Pose** Tadasana
Standing Forward Bend Uttanasana
Inhale into **Plank Pose** Kumbhakasana - deep breath in plank.
Exhale, Drop knees chest chin into **Cobra Pose** Bhujangasana (boo-jang-GAHS-uh-nah)
Hug elbows in, Press down through tops of feet. Inhale gently lift head and chest, shoulders back, heart forward. Gaze to the floor or up to the sky.

Chest and head up breathe into **Upward Dog** Urdhva Mukha Svanasana (OORD-vah MOO-kah shvon-AHS-anna) squeeze buttocks and legs together.
Push back into **Child's Pose** Balasana (bah-LAHS-ah-nuh)**,** arms extended, forehead on mat. Stay here breathing, allow your body to sink.

Inhale into **Table** Bharmanasana
Dancing Cat Utthita Cakravākāsana (oo-TEE-tah Cha-kravak-AHS-uh-nuh)
Extend RIGHT leg up, arch back, and exhale bringing knee to nose
Repeat dancing cat with right leg X 3
After last leg extention, Move RIGHT knee between arms and hands into
Pigeon Pose Eka Pada Rajakapotasana (EHK-a-PHOD-a-RHAH-ja-KAH-pot-AHS-uh-nah)
Lengthen through the spine, lengthen thighs away from each other, tailbone extends back, breastbone extends forward.
Hands on mat beside the knees, fold over the front leg, place forehead to mat, and extend arms all the way forward, relaxing the shoulders.
Pause for 5 counts of breath
Back to **Table** Bharmanasana
Dancing Cat Utthita Cakravākāsana
Extend LEFT leg up, arch back, and exhale bringing knee to nose
Repeat dancing cat with left leg X 3
After last leg extention, Move LEFT knee between arms and hands into
Pigeon Pose Eka Pada Rajakapotasana
Lengthen through the spine, lengthen thighs away from each other, tailbone extends back, breastbone extends forward.

Hands on mat beside the knees, fold over the front leg, place forehead to mat, and extend arms all the way forward, relaxing the shoulders.
Pause for 5 counts of breath

Lift head up and slowly shift the weight of the body to the front placing hands and forearms flat on the mat. Elbows beneath shoulders.
Tuck toes under and lift into **Dolphin Plank** Makara Adho Mukha Svanasana (mah-KAH-rah AH-doh MOO-kah shva-NAH-sun-uh)
Pause and take 3 breaths
Then raise the pelvis skyward for **Dolphin Pose** Makarasana (makar-AHS-uh-nuh)
Pause and take 3 breaths

Place knees down to prepare for Inversion:
Headstand Sirsasana (sheer-SHAH-sahn-ah)
Option using wall: Imagine holding a tennis ball between your palms. Come to all fours and place your forearms on the mat. Place the crown of head at the base of palms. Tuck toes under to lift your lower body. Have your arms and head about 5 inches from a wall and start to walk your feet up so your hips come over your shoulders, lower back comes to the wall and straiten the legs. Press firmly in to your forearms and outer wrists and engaging your core. Hold for at least 5 breath counts and gently lower down to the mat.

Child's Pose Balasana (bah-LAHS-ah-nuh)
Extend arms out, melt heart down, place forehead to mat, knees apart
Pause for 7 breath counts

Lay on the back with soles of the feet on the floor.
Inhale chest up and pelvis up into **Bridge Pose** Setu Bahdha Sarvangasana (SAY-too-BAHN-duh Shar-vahn-GAHS-ah-nuh)
*You can place a block beneath your lower back/low waist band area for support. Changing the height of the block can also improve flexibility and increase the effectiveness of the posture.
Exhale pelvis down, inhale up
Repeat Bridge x 3

Move to **Easy Pose** Sukasana
Shoulder releases inhale up and exhale down, keep neck relaxed. X 3
Slowly move left ear to left shoulder, stretching the right side of the neck. Back to center.
Slowly move right ear to right shoulder, stretching the left side of the neck. Back to center.
Gently take the head all the way back. Move the head into a full circle.
Then rotate the opposite way.

Relaxation Pose Savasana (sha-VAHS-ah-nuh)
Moving onto the back. Allow legs and feet to naturally fall to the sides.
Eyes closed and relaxed.
Soften your face. Part lips slightly. Bring your awareness to the breath.

Closing Meditation
yoga nidra journey of sensation
(Guided Savasana)

Let your body sink into the floor. Get comfortable.
Shift and move a little to let your body settle deeper into the ground.
Be comforted that at this time, everything is ok.
Nothing else matters right now. Everything is okay.
Allow yourself to simply feel your body and listen.
Do not worry or become agitated if you do not hear everything I say.
It is natural to flow in and out of conscious hearing. The deepest part of you, your core self, is always listening. Whatever you experience today, this practice will still work. So, there is no way to do this wrong.

You are in a safe environment, a protected space. Come into stillness and remain still for deep rest and deep nourishment, feel your natural breath. Allow your bones to become heavy. Feel them sinking into the earth.
Create a Sankalpa (sun-KULL-puh), an intention or affirmation based on your heart's longing. Think of this positive statement in the present tense, as though it's already happening.
For example, "I flow through life with ease and peace, I am relaxed".
Think of your intention/Sankalpa.
State it three times in your mind as though it is already happening.

Allow your awareness to travel through your head now on a journey of sensation.
Simply feel each part as it is mentioned, and without moving, remain still.
Feel and relax your mouth. Feel and relax your jaw, lips, upper lip, lower lip, notice where the lips touch, feel the inside of the mouth, roof, under tongue, teeth and gums, tongue, notice sense of taste in the mouth. Notice again the sensation of cool air passing through your nostrils and nasal passage. Feel your inner cheeks. Relax you eye sockets down. Feel them heavy. Bring your attention to the space between your eyes. Relax your forehead. Relax your inner ears, your outer ears. Feel the crown of your head and imagine the space of your brain. Feel into that space with your intention/Sankalpa.
Now feel the entire head together as a whole, feel this sensation, this energy, as radiant vibration.

Notice the breath again. After 5 counts of breath, let your eyes open, gently roll to your side and come up to a seated position.

Hands together at heart center. Namaste

Move Chill Yoga
Portable Yoga Class Plan 2
journey

Staff Pose
Seated twist with legs extended
Staff Pose stretches
Diamond Pose to **Rabbit Pose** stretch **x 3**
Sun Salutation A x 3
- Mountain pose
- Upward salute
- Standing forward fold
- Half forward fold
- High plank pose
- Upward-facing dog
- Downward-facing dog
- Half forward fold
- Standing forward fold
- Upward salute
- Mountain pose

Table Pose
Downward Dog/Plank x 3
Mountain/Forward bends
Standing Side Bends with interlaced fingers

Triangle Pose RIGHT x 2	**Triangle Pose LEFT x 2**
Supported Side Stretch	**Supported Side Stretch**
Tree RIGHT Leg	**Tree LEFT leg**
Mountain	**Mountain**

(option for group: Forest)
Mountain
Standing Forward Bend
Plank Pose
Cobra Pose
Upward Dog
Child's Pose

Table Pose	**Table Pose**
Dancing Cat RIGHT leg	**Dancing Cat LEFT leg**
Pigeon Pose	**Pigeon Pose**
Table Pose	

Dolphin Plank
Dolphin Pose
Headstand – wall option
Child's Pose
Bridge x 3
Easy Pose Shoulder releases
Relaxation Pose

color the mind

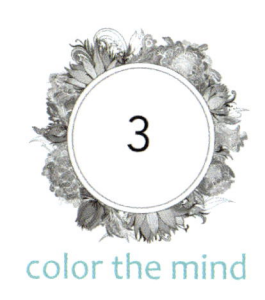

Opening Meditation
good feeling color

Choose a comfortable seat.
Release your weight down into the earth. Feel the tongue soft in the mouth, jaw lightly parted and relaxed.
Hear the sound of your own breathing. Practice an audible breath, meaning allow yourself to hear the hollow sound in your throat as you breathe in and out.

Think of your favorite color.
A good feeling color. Inhale in this color.
Exhale a slightly darker version of this color, pushing out anything you no longer need.
Again, inhaler your good feeling color, and on the exhale, a slightly darker shade takes everything you no longer need out of the body.
Think about your color. What does this color look like? It is vibrant or soft?
Think about what would this color smell like?

Now Imagine the Full Moon above in this color.
Imagine the light of this moon in this color flowing down so you're bathing in the light and the glow of this colored moon.
Allow this glow to flow into your heart, moving through your body.
Down the legs, down the arms into the toes and fingertips.

Invite in the possibility that anything is possible.
Exhale and release a little bit more of anything else you no longer need.
Continue to inhale your color as you feel the moon's glow shining on you.
Let the physical body feel light. Your energy is lighter.
And now your mind feels lighter.

Begin in **Child's Pose** Balasana (bah-LAHS-ah-nuh)
Extend arms out forward, melt heart down, place forehead to mat, knees apart.
Pause here and breathe for 5-10 breath counts

Move to lay on your front body for **Locust Pose** Shalabasana (sha-la-BAHS-ah-nuh)
Big toes lifted and touching, arms stretched out in front, arch your back. Lift your heart and gaze to the front of the space. If you can, lift your feet, legs, and thighs. Lifting through all limbs and lengthening the entire body.
Hold for 3 breath counts. Release down
Repeat x 2

Lower elbows to the floor for **Dolphin Pose** Makarasana (makar-AHS-uh-nuh)
Elbows beneath shoulders, forearms parallel, tuck toes and raise pelvis skyward. Straighten the legs.
Press the palms into the mat and lift into **Downward Dog** Adho Mukha Svanasana (AH-doh MOO-kah-shvah-Nahs-ana)
Raise pelvis skyward, pressing through all 10 fingers and palms. Head and neck are relaxed. Gaze at the core.
Release the kness down and move through **Upward Dog** Urdhva Mukha Svanasana (OORD-vah MOO-kah shvon-AHS-anna) Tops of the feet pressing into the floor, straighten your arms and simultaneously lift your torso up and your legs a few inches off the floor on an inhalation.
Tuck toes and push back to **Plank Pose** Kumbhakasana (koom-bahk-AHS-uh-nuh)
Lower down to the floor and again into **Locust Pose** Shalabasana
Big toes lifted and touching, arms stretched out in front, arch your back. Lift your heart and gaze to the front of the space. If you can, lift your feet, legs, and thighs. Lifting through all limbs and lengthening the body.
Hold for 3 breath counts. Release down.
Repeat x 2

Push into **Downward Dog** Adho Mukha Svanasana
Raise pelvis skyward, pressing through all 10 fingers and palms. Head is relaxed. Gaze at the core.
Release the knees down and move through **Upward Dog** Urdhva Mukha Svanasana
Tops of the feet pressing into the floor, straighten your arms and simultaneously lift your torso up and your legs a few inches off the floor on an inhalation.

Up into **Down Dog Split RIGHT LEG** Tri Pada Adho Mukha Svanasana (Tri Pada AH-doh MOO-kah-shvah-Nahs-ana)
Right leg lifts back and skyward, then knee to nose and place the right foot between hands into **High Lunge** arms all the way up
Place right hand on right hip, place the left hand on the floor next to the right foot
Twisting Lunge, raise right arm up skyward
Drop left knee, drop hips, and place both hands on the floor at your sides
Straiten right leg in front. Push back to a **Hamstring stretch**,
leaning back on the left leg

Back to **Downward Dog** Adho Mukha Svanasana
Upward Dog Urdhva Mukha Svanasana
Down Dog Split LEFT LEG Tri Pada Adho Mukha Svanasana
Left leg lifts back and skyward, then knee to nose and place the left foot between hands

High Lunge arms all the way up
Place left hand on left hip, place the right hand on the floor next to the left foot
Twisting Lunge, raise left arm up skyward
Drop right knee, drop hips, and place both hands on the floor at your sides
Straiten left leg in front. Push back to a **Hamstring stretch**,
leaning back on the right leg

Back to **Downward Dog** Adho Mukha Svanasana
Upward Dog Urdhva Mukha Svanasana

Stand in **Mountain Pose** Tadasana (Ta-DAHS-un-nah) feeling grounded through the feet
Standing forward Bend Uttanasana (OO-tan-AHS-un-nah)
into **Ragdoll** Uttanasana variation micro-bend the knees, head heavy, back of neck long, grab opposite elbows. Imagine the tension leaving your lower back

Back up to **Mountain Pose** Tadasana
Standing Forward Bend Uttanasana
Walk feet back to **Downward Dog** Adho Mukha Svanasana
Hold and breathe for 5 counts
Upward Dog Urdhva Mukha Svanasana
Back to **Downward Dog** Adho Mukha Svanasana
Stand into **Chair Pose** Utkatasana (OOT-kuh-TAHS-uh-nuh) Heart forward, weight to your heels, arms all the way up. Bend knees as if you are sitting in a chair. *You can place a block at it's narrowest width between your knees to increase strength in the abdominals and inner thighs.
Utkatasana means awkward chair. If you feel awkward, you are doing it correctly.
Repeat:
Mountain Pose Tadasana
Downward Dog Adho Mukha Svanasana
Upward Dog Urdhva Mukha Svanasana
Chair Pose Utkatasana

Downward Dog Adho Mukha Svanasana
Upward Dog Urdhva Mukha Svanasana
Down Dog Split RIGHT Tri Pada Adho Mukha Svanasana
Right leg lifts up and skyward, then steps between hands
Warrior I Virabhadrasana I (Veer-ah-bah-DRAHS-ana) Pivot on the ball of your back foot and drop your heel to the floor with your toes turned out about 45 degrees from the heel. Bend your front knee directly over the ankle so that the thigh is parallel to the floor. Rise to standing, bringing your arms out to the side and up toward the ceiling. Chest stays open as you come into a slight backbend. Touch palms overhead or keep arms parallel pointing upward. Hips pointing forward.

Extend arms out to a T into **Warrior II** Virabhadrasana II Gaze is forward. Shoulders down and relaxed. Breathe.

Cartwheel hands down to **Plank Pose** Kumbhakasana
Upward Dog Urdhva Mukha Svanasana
Down Dog Split LEFT Tri Pada Adho Mukha Svanasana
Left leg lifts up and skyward, then steps between hands
Warrior I Virabhadrasana I
Warrior II Virabhadrasana II

Cartwheel hands down to **Plank Pose** Kumbhakasana
Upward Dog Urdhva Mukha Svanasana

Downward Dog Split RIGHT Tri Pada Adho Mukha Svanasana
Right leg lifts, then steps between hands
Warrior I Virabhadrasana I
Warrior II Virabhadrasana II
Reverse Warrior Viparita Virabhadrasana (VIP-uh-REE-tuh veer-uh-buh-DRAHS-uh-nuh)
Drop your left hand to the back of your left thigh. On an inhalation, lift your right arm straight up, reaching your fingertips toward the ceiling. Your right bicep should be next to your right ear.
Keep your front knee bent and your hips sinking low as you lengthen through the sides of your waist. Slide your back hand further down your leg and come into a slight backbend.
Tilt your head slightly and bring your gaze to your right hand's fingertips.
Keep your shoulders relaxed, chest lifting, and the sides of your waist long.
Hold for 7 breath counts.
Move back up to **Warrior II** Virabhadrasana II

Cartwheel hands down **Plank Pose** Kumbhakasana
Upward Dog Urdhva Mukha Svanasana

Downward Dog Split LEFT Tri Pada Adho Mukha Svanasana
Left leg lifts, then steps between hands
Warrior I Virabhadrasana I
Warrior II Virabhadrasana II
Reverse Warrior Viparita Virabhadrasana
Drop your right hand to the back of your right thigh. On an inhalation, lift your left arm straight up, reaching your fingertips toward the ceiling. Your left bicep should be next to your left ear.
Keep your front knee bent and your hips sinking low as you lengthen through the sides of your waist. Slide your back hand further down your leg and come into a slight backbend.
Tilt your head slightly and bring your gaze to your left hand's fingertips.
Keep your shoulders relaxed, chest lifting, and the sides of your waist long.
Hold for 7 breath counts.
Move back up to **Warrior II** Virabhadrasana II

Cartwheel hands down **Plank Pose** Kumbhakasana
Upward Dog Urdhva Mukha Svanasana

Downward Dog Adho Mukha Svanasana
Walk feet up to **Mountain Pose** Tadasana
Sit into **Chair Pose** Utkatasana Extend arms all the way up, or keep palms together at heart center.
Move into **1-legged Chair Pose** RIGHT Eka Pada Utkatasana
(Eeka-pah-duh Oot-Kah –TAS –uh-nah)
Hugging in the right leg, and crossing it over the left knee, Bend your left knee as if sitting. Pause. Now straiten left leg.
With left foot planted firmly into mat, raise RIGHT leg into **Tree Pose**
Vrksasana (vrik-SHAH-suh-nuh) arms up and out, find an un-moving or **drishti** point to focus your gaze and help with balance.

Return to **Mountain Pose** Tadasana
Sit into **Chair Pose** Utkatasana Extend arms all the way up, or keep palms together at heart center.
Move into **1 legged Chair** LEFT Eka Pada Utkatasana
Hugging in the left leg, and crossing it over the right knee, Bend your right knee as if sitting. Pause. Now straiten right leg.
With right foot planted firmly into mat, raise LEFT leg into **Tree Pose** Vrksasana
arms up and out, find an un-moving or **drishti** point to focus your gaze and help with balance.

Back to **Mountain Pose** Tadasana
Sit down into **Staff Pose** Dandasana (dan-DAHS-ah-nah)
Lift arms all the way up, Lift chest and fold forward over your legs with a flat back
Repeat x 2

Move into **Child's Pose** Balasana
Push your seat back, extend arms out, melt heart down onto mat, place forehead to mat, knees apart. Pause for 3 breath counts

Come up to sit on the heels for **Camel Pose** Ustrasana (oosh-TRAHS-ah-nah)
Kneel upward with thighs perpendicular to the floor. Plant your shin bones into the mat, Lift pelvis up and bend backwards while exhaling slowly. Maintaining length in the body, push pelvis forward as you place hands on lower back. Head moves back.
To go deeper, extend arms down onto heels one by one pressing palms against the heels.

Sit for **Cobbler's Pose/Bound Ankle Pose** Baddha Konasana
(BAH-duh cone-AHS-uh-nuh)
*Place blocks beneath your knees for additional support. Soles of the feet together, let knees drop to both sides. Clasp big toes with thumb and first finger. Extend the length of your entire spine skyward. Hold for 5 counts of breath.

Lift feet up, knees bent, and balance into **Boat Pose** Navasana (na-VAHS-ah-nuh)
Straiten your legs if you can, keep torso upright, creating a V shape with the body. Roll shoulders back and straiten arms parallel to the floor. Balancing on the sit bones, hold for 5 breath counts.

Roll back onto the floor for
Happy Baby Pose Ananda Balasana (a-NAN-da ba-LAHS-ah-nah)
Exhale and bend knees in to your core. Grip outsides of feet, open knees slightly wider than torso and bring them up towards your armpits. Flex the feet.
Sink into the posture, taking your time. Breathe and hold.

Place the soles of the feet on the floor.
Half Bridge Ardha Setu Bandha Sarvangasana
(ahr-dah SAY-too-BAHN-duh Shar-vahn-GAHS-ah-nuh)
Come up to your elbows and forearms. Inhale chest up and pelvis up. Pushing into the forearms. Lift and straiten one leg upward and pause. Lift and straiten the other leg upward and pause.

Hug knees into chest.
Supported Shoulderstand Salamba Sarvangasana
(sa-LAM-bah SAR-vahn-GAHS-ah-nah)
Roll legs overhead, roll hips up and bring the knees into the chest hands on the back.
Lift and support with your arms. Straighten and extend legs skyward.
Pause and hold for 5 breath counts.
Continue on rolling the legs and feet back towards the opposite wall for
Plough Pose Halasana (ha-LAHS-ah-nah) guiding the body with your arms and hands.
Feet/toes touch the floor over your head. Hold.

Roll all the way down flat on the backbody for
Relaxation Pose Savasana (sha-VAHS-ah-nuh)
Feel your body on the mat. Let gravity take over and relax.

Closing Meditation
balancing your chakras in a color bath

This color meditation will help bring in peace and bring in the feeling of ease. Surrounding ourselves in light and sharing of light will assist in how people and the universe respond to you.

Take a deep breath in through your nose, and exhale out through your mouth.
Do this three times.

Picture a white light of universal love swirling around you in a circular motion, starting at your feet, and moving up towards your head. Picture this motion of white light going around you three times, each time starting at the bottom of your feet and moving upwards.

Next, picture your **crown chakra** at the very top of your head. Imagine a purple light swirling around in a circular motion swirling down toward your feet and back up. Purple brings in spirit.

Now move to the area on the forehead which is the **third-eye chakra**, your intuitive area. Picture an indigo color light in a circular motion and swirl it around your body down to your feet and back up to your head.

Next is the **throat chakra**, throat area which holds anger and the ability to speak up for oneself. Picture a light blue light swirling around your body to your feet and back up again to your head.

The chest area, which is known as the **heart chakra**, the center of love for self, and being able to love. This color is pink or green. Pick one of the colors and picture it moving swirl it around your body and down to your feet and back up to your head.

The **diaphragm chakra**, located right below your breastbone or in the stomach area is the color of yellow, and relates to emotional issues, once again picture the yellow light swirl it around your body and down to your feet and back up to your head.

The **belly chakra** color is orange, this relates to sexuality, imagine the swirl of color around your body, swirling up to the head and down the body.

Lastly the **root chakra** color is red, and located in the pelvic area, this relates to safety and security and grounding in all aspects of life.
Swirl the red light in the chakra area and then up and down the body.

If you are laying in **Relaxation Pose** Savasana, slowly come up to sit into
Easy Pose Sukasana.

Let your eyes float open. Hands at heart center. Namaste.

Move Chill Yoga
Portable Yoga Class Plan 3
color the mind

Child's Pose
Locust Pose x 2
Dolphin Pose
Downward Dog
Upward Dog
Plank
Locust Pose x 2
Downward Dog
Upward Dog

Downward Dog Split RIGHT leg	Downward Dog Split LEFT leg
High Lunge to Twisting Lunge	High Lunge to Twisting Lunge
Hamstring Stretch	Hamstring Stretch
Downward Dog	Downward Dog
Upward Dog	Upward Dog

Mountain/Forward bend and Ragdoll
Mountain/Standing forward bend
Downward Dog
Upward Dog
Downward Dog
Chair Pose
Mountain Pose/Standing Forward bend
Downward Dog
Upward Dog
Chair Pose
Downward Dog
Upward Dog

Downward Dog Split RIGHT	Downward Dog Split LEFT
Warrior I to Warrior II	Warrior I to Warrior II
Plank Pose	Plank Pose
Upward Dog	Upward Dog
Downward Dog Split RIGHT	Downward Dog Split LEFT
Warrior I to Warrior II	Warrior I to Warrior II
Reverse Warrior	Reverse Warrior
Warrior II	Warrior II
Plank Pose	Plank Pose
Upward Dog	Upward Dog

Downward Dog

Mountain Pose	Mountain Pose
Chair Pose	Chair Pose
1-Legged Chair RIGHT	1-Legged Chair LEFT
Tree RIGHT leg	Tree LEFT leg

Mountain Pose
Staff Pose stretches x 2
Child's Pose
Camel Pose
Cobbler's Pose
Boat Pose
Happy Baby Pose
Half Bridge lift RIGHT leg then LEFT
Supported Shoulderstand
Plough
Relaxation Pose

4

living in the moment

Opening Meditation
anchoring into the present

Sit in **Easy Pose** Sukhasana (Soo- KAHS-uh-nah)

The roots of a large tree spread deep underground, anchoring the tree into the earth. Use your mind to imagine roots, going down from your body plunging into the depths of the planet and spreading out, just like the roots of that tree.

Envision the strength of the roots extending downwards below the surface, broadening from the base of your spine.
These roots enable you to draw into your body the positive frequency of earth and ground you in the present moment.

Feel the awareness of the planet deep below the surface flooding into your space. Imagine the strong roots that are beginning to entwine with the waters inside the planet's core. These waters represent the unconditional love radiating from the plant, and the healing nature of allowing what IS.

Take a deep breath in. Envision yourself as a budding rose waiting for food and nurturing from nature.
The rose allows into now and into the power of the moment. The rose trusts the sun will shine for it to sprout, and trusts the rain will arrive and provide the adequate balance of water for growth.

When you entwine with the present moment, and resonate with the workings of the universe, you become the most central and most significant rendering of life.
You become just like that rose.

Continue to breathe and relax in **Easy Pose** Sukasana
Neck half circles: Bring your chin to your chest. Revolve the neck to the left. Bring the chin back to center and down to the chest again. Revolve the neck to the right.
Neck full circles: Now gently rotate the neck all the way around to the left. And then all the way around to the right.
Shoulder rolls: Inhale rolling the shoulders forward 3 times.
Exhale rolling the shoulders backward 3 times.

Move to **Table Pose** Bharmanasana (Bar-man-AHS-un-nah)
Place arms directly under shoulders, extend the neck and allow the back to be flat. Press the tail bone towards the back wall, and the crown of the head towards the front wall to lengthen the spine.
Into **Balancing Table** variation Dandayamna Bharmanasana (dan-day-AHM-na Bar-man-AHS-ah-nah)
Extend the RIGHT leg back to hip level and bend the back knee upwards to 90 degree angle with the sole of foot to sky. Pull low belly in toward your back. Allow shoulder blades to soften back and down. Extend left arm out and reach.
Push up to **Revolved Downward Dog** RIGHT Parivrtta Adho Mukha Svanasana (PAHR-ee-VREE-tah Ah-doh MOO-kuh shvan-AHS-uh-nuh)
In Downward Dog, reach the right hand around to the outer left calf muscle for the twist. Breathe and hold.
Move to **Child's Pose** Balasana (bah-LAHS-uh-nuh)
Keeping knees wide, keep big toes touching. Drape your torso between your thighs. Allow forehead to come to floor. Keep arms long and extended, palms facing down. Lengthen from hips. Sink into the posture.

Back to **Table Pose** Bharmanasana
Into **Balancing Table** variation Dandayamna Bharmanasana
Extend the LEFT leg back to hip level and bend the back knee upwards to 90 degree angle with the sole of foot to sky. Pull low belly in toward your back. Allow shoulder blades to soften back and down. Extend right arm out and reach.
Push up to **Revolved Downward Dog** LEFT Parivrtta Adho Mukha Svanasana
In Downward Dog, reach the left hand around to the outer right calf muscle for the twist.
Move to **Child's Pose** Balasana
Keeping knees wide, keep big toes touching. Drape your torso between your thighs. Allow forehead to come to floor. Keep arms long and extended, palms facing down. Lengthen from hips. Sink into the posture.

Come up to a kneel for **Camel Pose** Ustrasana (oosh-TRAHS-ah-nah)
Kneel upward with thighs perpendicular to the floor. Plant your shin bones into the mat, Lift pelvis up and bend backwards while exhaling slowly. Maintaining length in the body, push pelvis forward as you place hands on lower back. Head moves back. To go deeper, extend arms one by one pressing palms against heels.

Gate Pose RIGHT Parighasana (pah-ri-GAHS-ah-nuh)
Step RIGHT leg out to the side, rest the right hand on outstretched thigh. Inhale reach left arm up. Exhale leaning to the right for the side stretch.

Move back to **Table Pose** Bharmanasana (Bar-man-AHS-un-nah)
Press the tail bone towards the back wall and the crown of the head towards the front wall to lengthen the spine.
Push up to **Revolved Downward Dog** RIGHT Parivrtta Adho Mukha Svanasana
In Downward Dog, reach the right hand around to the outer left calf muscle for the twist.
Back to **Camel Pose** Ustrasana (oosh-TRAHS-ah-nah)
Try for a bit more length this time. Lift pelvis up and bend backwards while exhaling slowly. Maintaining length in the body, push pelvis forward as you place hands on lower back. Head moves back.
To go deeper, extend arms one by one pressing palms against heels.
Gate Pose LEFT Parighasana (pah-ri-GAHS-ah-nuh)
Step LEFT leg out to the side, rest the left hand on outstretched thigh. Inhale reach right arm up. Exhale leaning to the right for the side stretch.
Move back to **Table Pose** Bharmanasana (Bar-man-AHS-un-nah)
Press the tail bone towards the back wall and the crown of the head towards the front wall to lengthen the spine.
Push up to **Revolved Downward Dog** LEFT Parivrtta Adho Mukha Svanasana
In Downward Dog, reach the left hand around to the outer right calf muscle for the twist.

Mountain Pose Tadasana (Ta-DAHS-un-nah)
Stand firm and grounded through the feet. Hands at your sides.
Standing Forward Bend Uttanasana (OO-tan-AHS-un-nah)
Allow gravity to pull you down with a flat back.
Bending your knees, raise the arms up into **Chair Pose** Utkatasana (OOT-kuh-TAHS-uh-nuh) Heart forward, weight to your heels, arms all the way up. Bend knees as if you are sitting in a chair. Utkatasana means awkward chair. If you feel awkward, you are doing it correctly.
Open the RIGHT leg back for **Warrior I** Virabhadrasana I (Veer-ah-bah-DRAHS-ana)
Pivot on the ball of your back foot and drop your heel to the floor with your toes turned out about 45 degrees from the heel. Bend your front knee directly over the ankle so that the thigh is parallel to the floor. Rise to standing, bringing your arms out to the side and up toward the ceiling. Chest stays open as you come into a slight backbend. Touch palms together overhead. Hips pointing forward.
Slide the prayer down to your chest, into **Crescent Lunge Twist** RIGHT Anjaneyasana (AHN-jah-nay-AHS-uh-nuh)
Twist the body bringing the right elbow to left knee and twist to the left side space. Reach your heart skyward, and gaze up over the left shoulder.
Release hands to the front of the mat and into **Forward Fold** Uttanasana
Jump or walk back to **Plank Pose** Kumbhakasana (koom-bahk-AHS-uh-nuh)
Lower knees, chest, chin, for **Cobra Pose** Bhujangasana (boo-jang-GAHS-uh-nah)
Hug elbows in, Press down through tops of feet. Inhale gently lift head and chest, shoulders back, heart forward. Gaze to the floor or up to the sky.

Move through **Upward Dog** Urdhva Mukha Svanasana
Tops of the feet pressing into the floor, straighten your arms and simultaneously lift your torso up and your legs a few inches off the floor on an inhalation.
Tuck toes and push back to **Downward Dog** Adho Mukha Svanasana (AH-doh MOO-kah-shvah-Nahs-ana)
Deep breath - All 10 fingers and palms pressing into mat, hips up as if a string is pulling up the hips, gaze at belly button
Find stillness here.

Mountain Pose Tadasana
Stand firm and grounded through the feet. Hands at your sides.
Standing Forward Bend Uttanasana
Allow gravity to pull you down with a flat back.
Bending your knees, raise the arms up into **Chair Pose** Utkatasana
Heart forward, weight to your heels, arms all the way up. Bend knees as if you are sitting in a chair.
Open the LEFT leg back for **Warrior I** Virabhadrasana I (Veer-ah-bah-DRAHS-ana)
Pivot on the ball of your back foot and drop your heel to the floor with your toes turned out about 45 degrees from the heel. Bend your front knee directly over the ankle so that the thigh is parallel to the floor. Rise to standing, bringing your arms out to the side and up toward the ceiling. Chest stays open as you come into a slight backbend. Touch palms together overhead. Hips pointing forward.
Slide the prayer down to your chest, into **Crescent Lunge Twist** LEFT Anjaneyasana
Twist the body bringing the left elbow to right knee and twist to the right side space. Reach your heart skyward, and gaze up over the right shoulder.
Release to **Forward Fold** Uttanasana
Jump or walk back to **Plank Pose** Kumbhakasana
Lower knees, chest, chin, for **Cobra Pose** Bhujangasana (boo-jang-GAHS-uh-nah)
Hug elbows in, Press down through tops of feet. Inhale gently lift head and chest, shoulders back, heart forward. Gaze to the floor or up to the sky.
Move through **Upward Dog** Urdhva Mukha Svanasana
Tops of the feet pressing into the floor, straighten your arms and simultaneously lift your torso up and your legs a few inches off the floor on an inhalation.
Tuck toes and push back to
Downward Dog Adho Mukha Svanasana
Deep breath - All 10 fingers and palms pressing into mat, hips up as if a string is pulling up the hips, gaze at belly button
Find stillness.

Walk up to **Mountain Pose** Tadasana
Stand firm and grounded through the feet.
Hands at heart center.
Sit into **Chair Pose** Utkatasana Hands together at heart center
Bend into **Yogi Squat** Malasana (ma-LAHS-ah-nuh) Hands at heart center.
Bend the knees and lower your tailbone toward the floor to come into a squat. The toes will want to want to turn out and that's ok. Eventually, you're working toward keeping the feet closer to parallel.
From here, try to gently twist the core to the right, then to the left.

Come up to stand in **Mountain Pose** Tadasana
Hands at heart center. Pause here in **Equal Standing Balance** Samastitihi (Sa-mahs-TEE-tee-hee) **is an invitation to come into this moment, an opportunity to make the slate clean, to stand up and realign ourselves with balance. We become like a majestic mountain, rooted in the earth and totally still, present and magnificent. With total clarity, fully aware of this moment and of what IS.**
Relaxing the shoulders away from the ears. Be in the moment for 10 breath counts.

With LEFT foot planted firmly into the earth, move into **Tree pose** Vrksasana (vrik-SHAH-suh-nuh) lifting RIGHT Leg, Hands at heart, raise them up and out. Balance.
Transition to **King Dancer Pose** Natarajasana (NOT-ah-rahj-AHS-uh-nuh)
Bring your right heel toward your right buttock. Reach your right hand down and clasp your right foot's inner ankle. You can also loop a strap around the top of your right foot, and then hold onto the strap with your right hand. Reach your left arm overhead, pointing your fingertips toward the ceiling and facing your palm to the right.
Fix your gaze softly at a **drishti** point or unmoving point of focus. Make sure your left kneecap and toes point directly forward.
When you feel steady, begin to lift your right foot away from your body as you lean your torso slightly forward. Keep your chest lifted and continue reaching your left hand's fingertips up toward the ceiling. Raise your right foot as high as you can.
Come back to **Equal Standing Balance** Samastitihi
Open RIGHT leg back to **Triangle Pose** Utthita Trikonasana (oo-TEE-tah tree-koh-NAH-suh-nuh) Inhale arms up and tip forward like a teapot, chest open, left arm to left foot. Move as if you are standing between 2 panes of glass. Gaze upward, right arm is pointing up. Breathe.
Inhale come up keeping arms extend arms outward into a
Warrior II Virabhadrasana II (Veer-ah-bah-DRAHS-ana) stance. Arms out to the sides, bend the front knee and gaze forward. Relax shoulders down.
Frame the front foot, bringing both hands to the mat, and push to
Downward Dog Adho Mukha Svanasana Breathe and hold here.
Move to **Revolved Side Angle Pose** Parivrtta Parsvakonasana (PAHR-ee-VREE-tah PARZH-vuh-ko-NAHS-uh-nuh)
Bring left foot forward to the inside your left hand. Your toes should be in line with your fingers.
Bend your left knee so that your calf and thigh make a right angle with your thigh parallel to the floor.
Tuck the right toes and pivot on the ball of your right foot. Flatten the right hand to the floor under your right shoulder.
Twist your torso toward your left knee, opening the chest to the left side of the space. Lift your left arm up toward the ceiling. Bring your gaze up to the left hand.
Come up and move back into **Warrior II** Virabhadrasana II
Then, relax into **Equal Standing Balance** Samastitihi

With RIGHT foot planted firmly into the earth, move into **Tree pose** Vrksasana lifting LEFT Leg, Hands at heart, raise them up and out. Balance.
Transition to **King Dancer Pose** Natarajasana
Bring your left heel toward your left buttock. Reach your left hand down and clasp your left foot's inner ankle. You can also loop a strap around the top of your left foot, and then hold onto the strap with your left hand. Reach your right arm overhead, pointing your fingertips toward the ceiling and facing your palm to the left.
Fix your gaze softly at a **drishti** point or unmoving point of focus. Make sure your right kneecap and toes point directly forward.
When you feel steady, begin to lift your left foot away from your body as you lean your torso slightly forward. Keep your chest lifted and continue reaching your right hand's fingertips up toward the ceiling. Raise your left foot as high as you can.
Come back to **Equal Standing Balance** Samastitihi
Open LEFT leg back to **Triangle Pose** Utthita Trikonasana
(oo-TEE-tah tree-koh-NAH-suh-nuh) Inhale arms up and tip forward like a teapot, chest open, right arm to right foot. Move as if you are standing between 2 panes of glass. Gaze upward, left arm is pointing up. Breathe.
Inhale come up keeping arms extend arms outward into a
Warrior II Virabhadrasana II (Veer-ah-bah-DRAHS-ana) stance. Arms out to the sides, bend the front knee and gaze forward. Relax shoulders down.
Frame the front foot, bringing both hands to the mat, and push to
Downward Dog Adho Mukha Svanasana Breathe and hold here.
Move to **Revolved Side Angle Pose** Parivrtta Parsvakonasana
Bring right foot forward to the inside your right hand. Your toes should be in line with your fingers.
Bend your right knee so that your calf and thigh make a right angle with your thigh parallel to the floor.
Tuck the left toes and pivot on the ball of your left foot. Flatten the left hand to the floor under your left shoulder.
Twist your torso toward your right knee, opening the chest to the right side of the space. Lift your right arm up toward the ceiling. Bring your gaze up to the right hand.
Come up and move back to **Warrior II** Virabhadrasana II
Then, relax into **Equal Standing Balance** Samastitihi

Standing forward Bend Uttanasana (OO-tan-AHS-un-nah)
Fold over the legs with a flat back. Come up half way for a **Half Lift,** hands on the front thighs and **Fold Forward** Uttanasana

Jump or walk back to **Plank Pose** Kumbhakasana
Lower knees, chest, chin, for **Cobra Pose** Bhujangasana
Hug elbows in, Press down through tops of feet. Inhale gently lift head and chest, shoulders back, heart forward. Gaze to the floor or up to the sky.
move through **Upward Dog** Urdhva Mukha Svanasana
Tops of the feet pressing into the floor, straighten your arms and simultaneously lift your torso up and your legs a few inches off the floor on an inhalation.

Tuck toes and push back to **Downward Dog** Adho Mukha Svanasana
Deep breath - All 10 fingers and palms pressing into mat, hips up as if a string is pulling up the hips, gaze at belly button

Walk to front of mat and sit into **Staff Pose** Dandasana (dan-DAHS-ah-nah)
Seated Forward Fold Paschimottanasana (PAH-shee-moh-tun-AHS-uh-nuh)
Lengthen the tailbone away from the pelvis. Arms all the way up. Bend over the legs with a flat, strait back and reach for the sides of the feet with your hands. Thumbs on the inner soles, elbows fully extended. You can also loop a strap around the foot soles, and hold the strap firmly.
Come up and Repeat x 2

Place hands behind you, fingers pointing towards the body for
Reverse Plank Purvottanasana (PUR-voh-tun-AHS-uh-nuh) variation.
Strong through the arms and hands, engage the core and lift hips upward. Feel legs reaching away from the torso. Arms and shoulders away from ears. Gaze forward.
Bend the right leg, setting the sole of the foot to the floor underneath you.
Turn over to **Plank Pose** Kumbhakasana Breathe, and begin
Side Plank Pose Vasisthasana (vah-sish-TAHS-anna)
Keeping the left hand firm on the floor, lift your RIGHT hand up slowly as you open up your torso to the right. As you turn your torso, align the shoulders skyward. Place your right hand on your hip, then straiten and raise it up. Try to straiten the right leg, bringing it even with the left.

Sit back into **Staff Pose** Dandasana (dan-DAHS-ah-nah)
Seated Forward Fold Paschimottanasana
Lengthen the tailbone away from the pelvis. Arms all the way up. Bend over the legs with a flat back and reach for the sides of the feet with your hands, thumbs on the inner soles, elbows fully extended. You can also loop a strap around the foot soles, and hold the strap firmly.
x 2

Place hands behind you, fingers pointing towards the body for
Reverse Plank Purvottanasana variation. Strong through the arms and hands, engage the core and lift hips upward. Feel legs reaching away from the torso. Arms and shoulders away from ears. Gaze forward.
Bend the left leg, setting the sole of the foot to the floor underneath you.
Turn over to **Plank Pose** Kumbhakasana Breathe, and begin
Side Plank Pose Vasisthasana
Keeping the right hand firm on the floor, lift your LEFT hand up slowly as you open up your torso to the left. As you turn your torso, align the shoulders skyward. Place your left hand on your hip, then straiten and raise it up. Try to straiten the left leg, bringing it even with the right.

Release back into **Staff Pose** Dandasana and walk up to **Mountain Pose** Tadasana
Jump or walk back to **Plank Pose** Kumbhakasana
Lower knees, chest, chin, for **Cobra Pose** Bhujangasana

Hug elbows in, Press down through tops of feet. Inhale gently lift head and chest, shoulders back, heart forward. Gaze to the floor or up to the sky.
move through **Upward Dog** Urdhva Mukha Svanasana
Tops of the feet pressing into the floor, straighten your arms and simultaneously lift your torso up and your legs a few inches off the floor on an inhalation.
Tuck toes and push back to
Downward Dog Adho Mukha Svanasana Deep breath - All 10 fingers and palms pressing into mat, hips up as if a string is pulling up the hips, gaze at belly button

Down Dog Split RIGHT LEG Tri Pada Adho Mukha Svanasana
(Tri Pada AH-doh MOO-kah-shvah-Nahs-ana)
Right leg lifts back and skyward, then knee to nose and place the right knee down on mat between hands
Pigeon Pose Eka Pada Rajakapotasana (EHK-a-PHOD-a-RHAH-ja-KAH-pot-AHS-uh-nah)
Lengthen through the spine, lengthen thighs away from each other, tailbone extends back, breastbone extends forward.
Hands on mat beside the knees, fold over leg, place forehead to mat, and extend arms all the way forward, relaxing the shoulders. Allow gravity, don't force the pose
Pause for 5 counts of breath.
Downward Dog Adho Mukha Svanasana
Raise pelvis skyward, pressing through all 10 fingers and palms. Head is relaxed. Gaze at the core. Move to **Plank Pose** Kumbhakasana Hold.
Knees Chest and Chin lower into **Cobra** Bhujangasana (boo-jang-GAHS-uh-nah)
Hug elbows in, Press down through tops of feet. Inhale gently lift head and chest, shoulders back, heart forward. Gaze to the floor or up to the sky.

Down Dog Split LEFT LEG Tri Pada Adho Mukha Svanasana
Left leg lifts back and skyward, then knee to nose and place the left knee down on mat between hands
Pigeon Pose Eka Pada Rajakapotasana Lengthen through the spine, lengthen thighs away from each other, tailbone extends back, breastbone extends forward.
Hands on mat beside the knees, fold over leg, place forehead to mat, and extend arms all the way forward, relaxing the shoulders. Allow gravity, don't force the pose
Pause for 5 counts of breath.
Downward Dog Adho Mukha Svanasana
Raise pelvis skyward, pressing through all 10 fingers and palms. Head is relaxed. Gaze at the core. Move to **Plank Pose** Kumbhakasana Hold.
Knees Chest and Chin lower into **Cobra** Bhujangasana (boo-jang-GAHS-uh-nah)
Hug elbows in, Press down through tops of feet. Inhale gently lift head and chest, shoulders back, heart forward. Gaze to the floor or up to the sky.

Light neck stretch: Lower to belly. Rest your right cheek to the mat. Lift the head and chest for a soft neck stretch. Place forehead on mat coming to center. Then left cheek to mat.
Lift the head and chest for a soft neck stretch.

Bring arms and hands to your sides for **Bow Pose** Dhanurasana
(DAHN-yoor-AHS-uh-nuh) Bend your knees. Bring your heels as close as you can to
your buttocks, keeping your knees hip-distance apart.
Reach back with both hands and hold onto your outer ankles.
On an inhalation, lift your heels up toward the ceiling, drawing your thighs up
and off the mat. Your head, chest, and upper torso will also lift off the mat.
Gaze forward and extend and lift a little higher.
Release down flat on the mat. Repeat x 2.

Push torso back and sit in **Yogi Squat** Malasana (Mah-LAHS-ah-nah)
to prepare for inversion: **Crow Pose** Bakasana (bah-KAHS-uh-nuh)
Bring your palms to the mat, shoulder-distance apart. Spread your fingers and
press evenly across both palms. Press your shins against the back of your upper
arms. Draw your knees in as close to your underarms as possible.
Lift onto the balls of your feet as you lean forward. Round your back and draw
your core in firmly. Look at the imaginary 12 o'clock spot on the floor in front of
you. *You can use a block between your hands and place your head on the
block for balance.
As you continue to lean forward, lift your feet off the floor and draw your heels
toward your buttocks. Try lifting one foot and then the other. Balance your
torso and legs on the back of your upper arms. Touch your big toes together.
Draw your belly in. Breathe steadily.
Advanced: Begin to straighten your elbows. Keep your knees and shins hugging
in tightly toward your armpits. Keep your forearms drawn firmly toward the
midline of your body.

Release to **Child's Pose** Balasana (bah-LAHS-ah-nuh)
Extend arms out, melt heart down, place forehead to mat, knees apart
Pause for 7 breath counts

Sit in **Lotus Pose** Padmasana (pahd-MAHS-ah-nah)
Bend your right knee and hug it to your chest. Then, bring your right ankle to
the crease of your left hip so the sole of your right foot faces the sky. The top
of your foot should rest on your hip crease.
Then, bend your left knee. Cross your left ankle over the top of your right shin.
The sole of your left foot should also face upwards, and the top of your foot
and ankle should rest on your hip crease.
Draw your knees as close together as possible. Press your groins toward the
floor and sit up straight.
Try **Elevated Lotus Posture** Utthita Padmasana (oo-tee-tah pahd-MAHS-ah-nah)
Place your palms on the ground next to your hips. Gradually and smoothly raise your
body above ground level so that your entire body weight rests on the palms of your
hands. Hold the breath in your lungs as long as you can hold this posture.
Release down and release the breath.

Extend legs and arms and lay flat for **Relaxation Pose** Savasana (sha-VAHS-ah-nuh)
Close the eyes and let gravity take over. Feel the back body on the mat. Breathe from
the belly.

Closing Meditation
the moment now
(Guided Savasana)

Make any adjustments to feel comfortable
As we rest and surrender, the mind stops to relax and let go
We are looking to swap out thinking to quality of feeling.
To come into presence, to come into right now.

Welcome in your experiences from today.
Notice some places in our body that feel tense, some are relaxed, and some feel nothing at all. Welcome it all in and just be with your physical self.
Feel your breathing entering and leaving

Feel how the mind focuses on the past or how things will be in the future
See what you can do to allow it all to be just as it is for a moment.
No need to try and make things better or find solutions – just allow what IS.

Bring your attention to relaxing various parts of the body, feel as though they are touched with a feather.
Relax in your mouth, the insides of the cheeks and the floor and roof of the mouth.
The teeth and gums. Your jaw, throat. Inside to the ears left and right.
Feel the gentle touch of air on your face.
Feel the air pass into the nostrils and inside the nose.
Bring your attention and relax the eyes deep in their sockets, eyebrows, forehead.
Sense through the very top of the head, sense through the back of the head, the back of the neck. Down and into the shoulders, shoulder blades. Relax them down and away from the ears. Melt the arms and the palms of the hands. See if you can sense into the palms of your hands.

Bring your attention to your lower back, side waists, hips,
Sense any currents from the hips to the legs and down to the feet.

Feel the space your body is in, the boundaries.
Give up the concept or thinking about where your body ends and the outer space around it begins. Allow this questioning to take you outside your body for a moment.
Floating here. Nothing to do. No where you need to be at the moment.
Just be here.
Feel how you are just living in the moment right now.
Find where you can bring this quality of being into every single day.

Find your way awake. Come up to a seated position, feeling well and happy.
Namaste

Move Chill Yoga
Portable Yoga Class Plan 4
living in the moment

Easy Pose – Neck circles/shoulder rolls
Table Pose to Balancing Table RIGHT leg
Revolved Downward Dog RIGHT leg
Child's Pose
Table Pose to Balancing Table LEFT leg
Revolved downward Dog LEFT leg
Child's Pose

Camel Pose
Gate Pose RIGHT leg
Table Pose
Revolved Downward Dog RIGHT leg

Camel Pose
Gate Pose LEFT leg
Table Pose
Revolved Downward Dog LEFT leg

Mountain Pose
Standing Forward Bend
Chair Pose
Warrior I, RIGHT leg back
Crescent Lunge Twist
Forward Fold
Plank Pose
Cobra Pose
Upward Dog
Downward Dog

Mountain Pose
Standing Forward Bend
Chair Pose
Warrior I, LEFT leg back
Crescent Lunge Twist
Forward Fold
Plank Pose
Cobra Pose
Upward Dog
Downward Dog

Mountain Pose
Chair Pose
Yogi Squat -
Mountain
Equal Standing Balance

Tree Pose RIGHT
King Dancer RIGHT
Equal Standing Balance
Triangle Pose – RIGHT leg back
Warrior II
Downward Dog
Revolved Side Angle
Warrior II
Equal Standing Balance

Tree Pose LEFT
King Dancer LEFT
Equal Standing Balance
Triangle Pose – LEFT leg back
Warrior II
Downward Dog
Revolved Side Angle
Warrior II
Equal Standing Balance

Standing Forward Bend – Half Lift
Forward Fold
Plank Pose
Cobra Pose
Upward Dog
Downward Dog

Staff Pose
Seated Forward Fold
Reverse Plank
Plank Pose
Side Plank RIGHT arm up

Staff Pose
Seated Forward Fold
Reverse Plank
Plank Pose
Side Plank LEFT arm up

Staff Pose
Mountain Pose
Plank Pose
Cobra Pose
Upward Dog
Downward Dog

Downward Dog Split RIGHT leg
Pigeon Pose RIGHT leg
Downward Dog
Plank Pose
Cobra Pose

Downward Dog Split LEFT leg
Pigeon Pose LEFT leg
Downward Dog
Plank Pose
Cobra Pose

Light Neck Stretch
Bow Pose
Yogi Squat
Crow Pose
Child's Pose
Lotus Pose into Elevated Lotus Pose
Relaxation Pose

5
power within

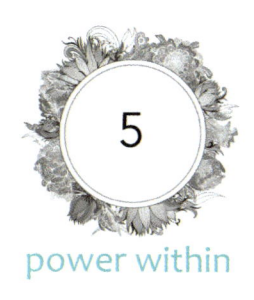

Opening Meditation
opposite sensations

Begin in **Easy Pose** Sukhasana (Soo- KAHS-uh-nah)
Lightness/Heaviness:
Imagine the whole body becoming light. As though your body could float away from the floor and toward the ceiling.
The head is light and weightless, the limbs are light and weightless, the torso is light and weightless, the whole body light and weightless.
You are rising higher and higher away from the floor.

Now, imagine your body becoming heavy.
Feel the heaviness in all parts of the body, each part is becoming heavier and heavier and heavier.
The head is heavy, the limbs are heavy, the torso is heavy, the whole body is heavy.
So heavy that it is sinking down into the floor.
Ask and notice - Is it possible to feel both the heaviness and lightness at the same time?

Cold/Hot:
Awaken the experience of cold in the body, the experience of chilly cold. Imagine being outside in winter without enough clothing. You feel this chill permeating your entire body.
Now, allow the sensation of warmth to spread throughout the entire body. Remember the feeling of heat in summer when you are out in the sun with no shade. You feel heat radiating onto your skin, heat all around the body.
Ask and notice - Is it possible for you to sense and feel both cold and hot at the same time?

Anxiety/Calm:
Recollect the experience of anxiety, intense anxiety, and worry. Feel this stress in your mind and body but do not concentrate on its source. Create the experience of anxiety as clearly as possible.
Now, allow the feeling of complete calm to envelop you. Breathe in even more calm. Manifest the experience of calm in your entire mind, body and emotions.
Lastly, try and recall both emotions at the same time

Breathe deeply. You are relaxed and aware, you are completely calm. Your mind has the power to feel and recall any emotion at any time. You may not have a choice with everything that happens in life, however, your mind has a choice with your emotions.

This practice emphasizes the use of blocks, and will take you through each posture using either 1 or 2 blocks.

Blocks can be helpful for both the beginner and seasoned yogi.
For beginners, yoga blocks can be used when the flexibility isn't quite there yet.
For more advanced yogis, they can help deepen postures. The key point to remember when you're using a block is to not sink or rest your hand on the block. Rather, keep the fingers spread, and use the hand propped up with the fingers. This engages the muscles in the hands and arms will help the body find a lift, which strengthens and lengthens.

Easy Pose Sukhasana Sit on 1 block, on its shortest height.
Table Pose Bharmanasana (Bar-man-AHS-un-nah)
Come to all fours with your shoulders stacked over your wrists, your hips stacked over your knees, and the tops of your feet relaxed down on the mat.
Slowly begin to walk your hands out in front of you, lowering your chest to the ground.
Extended Puppy Pose Uttana Shishosana (oo-tah-na Shish-AHS-uh-nuh)
Using 2 blocks on their shortest height, place them in front of you under your extended arms. Place 2 elbows and the back of the upper arms on the 2 blocks in front. Bring hands/palms together above the blocks. Allow your neck to relax and breathe into your back, lengthening your spine in opposite directions. Sink into the stretch here. Breathe.
Come to **Hero Pose** Vajrasana (vahj-RAHS-uh-nuh)
Sitting on the heels. Inhale arms all the way up. Bring hands down to heart center.
Push to **Downward Dog** Adho Mukha Svanasana (AH-doh MOO-kah-shvah-Nahs-ana)
Using 2 blocks in front on their shortest height, place hands on each block. This creates space in the upper body, especially in the shoulders and the neck. (the blocks can also help you transition/hop/glide from the back of the mat to the front of the mat) Lift your hips, let your neck be soft.
Transition to the top of the mat space into **Standing Forward Bend** Uttanasana (OO-tan-AHS-un-nah) - bend with a flat back, placing hands down to 2 blocks
Keep a flat back and come up to **Mountain Pose** Tadasana (Ta-DAHS-un-nah)
Standing forward Bend Uttanasana
　　　　　-Push the blocks off of the top of your mat for now-
RIGHT leg back into **High Lunge** Anjaneyasana (AHN-jah-nay-AHS-uh-nuh)
Balancing on the ball of your right foot, lift your heel and draw it forward so it aligns directly over your back toes. Reach arms up, squaring hips forward
Straighten your back leg completely.
Move to **High Plank Pose** Kumbhakasana (koom-bahk-AHS-uh-nuh) – make use of the muscles in the upper back. Engage the core. Maintain smooth even breaths.
Side Plank Vasistasana (VAH-shees-THAH-suh-nuh)
Bring RIGHT hand to middle of the mat and roll onto the side of the left foot. Raise the right knee strait up to the ceiling, keeping the feet in line with the lower leg. If you can, take the "peace" (first and middle) fingers to the big toe and straiten the leg skyward.
From here, **Wild Thing variation** Camatkarasana (cah-maht-kah-RAHS-anna)
Wild Thing is a lateral stretch, a backbend, and an amazing heart opener.
Lower and bring that right leg behind the body, lowering it to the floor. Allow yourself to flip into a gentle backbend. Reaching the right arm long and lifting the heart high.

From here, very gently move back to **High Plank Pose** Kumbhakasana lower down
Chaturanga Chaturanga Dandasana
(chah-tuur-ANGH-uh dahn-DAHS-uh-nuh)
Lift through your chest, keeping your shoulders in line with your elbows. Do not let your chest drop or sag toward the floor. Just lower down slowly. Keeping the elbows hugged along your ribcage, pointed toward your heels.
Fully engage your abdominal and leg muscles. If the full pose is too challenging right now, you can drop your knees. Then, lower your torso to hover an inch above the floor. This is **Half Chaturanga.**
Pause and lift into **Upward Dog** Urdhva Mukha Svanasana
(OORD-vah MOO-kah shvon-AHS-anna)
Straitening arms. Keep shoulders relaxed. Hold for 3 breaths
Push to **Downward Dog** Adho Mukha Svanasana
Deep breath - All 10 fingers and palms pressing into mat, hips up as if a string is pulling up the hips, gaze at belly button
Find stillness.

LEFT leg back into **High Lunge** Anjaneyasana
Balancing on the ball of your left foot, lift your heel and draw it forward so it aligns directly over your back toes. Reach arms up, squaring hips forward
Straighten your back leg completely.
Move to **High Plank Pose** Kumbhakasana
Side Plank Vasistasana – bring LEFT hand to middle of the mat and roll onto the side of the right foot. Raise the left knee strait up to the ceiling, keeping the feet in line with the lower leg. If you can, take the "peace" (first and middle) fingers to the big toe and straiten the leg skyward.
From here **Wild Thing variation** Camatkarasana lower and bring that left leg behind the body, lowering it to the floor. Allow yourself to flip into a gentle backbend. Reaching the left arm long and lifting the heart high.
From here, very gently move back to **High Plank Pose** Kumbhakasana
lower down **Chaturanga** Chaturanga Dandasana
Pause and lift into **Upward Dog** Urdhva Mukha Svanasana
(OORD-vah MOO-kah shvon-AHS-anna)
Straitening arms. Keep shoulders relaxed. Hold for 3 breaths
Downward Dog Adho Mukha Svanasana
Deep breath - All 10 fingers and palms pressing into mat, hips up as if a string is pulling up the hips, gaze at belly button
Find stillness

Walk feet to top of mat – **Standing forward Bend** Uttanasana
Up to **Mountain Pose** Tadasana
Down to **Downward Dog** Adho Mukha Svanasana
Down Dog Split RIGHT LEG Tri Pada Adho Mukha Svanasana
(Tri Pada Adho Mukha Svanasana)
Right leg extends towards the sky. Bring the right leg forward through the hands.
Right knee at 90 degree angle and come up for **Warrior I** Virabhadrasana I
(Veer-ah-bah-DRAHS-ana)

Arms strait up towards the sky. Create 1 long line of energy from your back heel through the tips of your fingers.

Interlace fingers behind you. **Devotional/Humble Warrior** Baddha Virabhadrasana (ba-DAH Veer-ah-bah-DRAHS-ana)
Inhale expanding chest and lungs. As you exhale, continue to keep your heart open and gently bow forward, while your arms extend backward and upward. The right shoulder may graze the right leg even further to the right as you release your pelvis and drop deeper into the pose.
As you come up, place blocks on the front corners of the top of mat on the tallest height, Move to **Warrior II** Virabhadrasana II
Arms out to a T, relax the shoulders down.
Glance to see your blocks are in place for **Half Moon Pose** Ardha Chandrasana (ARD-uh chan-DRAHS-uh-nuh)
Reach through your right hand. Shift your left hip back, and then fold sideways and forward at the hip. Rest your right hand's fingertips onto your block. Align your shoulders so your left shoulder is directly above your right shoulder.
Bring your left hand to rest on your left hip.
Straighten your right leg while simultaneously lifting your left leg. Work to bring the left leg parallel to the floor, or even higher than your hips.
Reach actively through your left heel. Take care to not lock the right leg's knee.
Stack top hip directly over your bottom hip, and open your torso to the left. Then extend your left arm and point your fingertips directly toward the sky. Balance.
Find a **drishti** point, or an unmoving point of focus.
Draw your shoulderblades firmly into your back. Lengthen your tailbone toward your left heel.
To release, lower your left leg as you exhale, and shift back to **Warrior II** Virabhadrasana II
Triangle Pose Utthita Trikonasana (oo-TEE-tah tree-koh-NAH-suh-nuh)
Keep the right foot out so your toes are pointing to the top of the mat, and straiten the front leg.
Your arms should be aligned directly over your legs. With your palms facing down, reach actively from fingertip to fingertip.
On an exhalation, reach through your right hand in the same direction as your right foot is pointed. Shift your left hip back and fold down at your right hip.
Keep your right ear, shoulder, and knee on the same plane (as if you are tipping like a teapot or moving within 2 panes of glass) Reach up with the left arm, fingertips reaching toward the sky. Align your shoulders so your left shoulder is directly above your right shoulder. Move the block directly next to and behind the right heel. As you tip down, place your right hand's fingertips on the block. Gaze up toward the sky.

Stand at the top of your mat **Mountain Pose** Tadasana
Place the RIGHT leg back about 3 to 4 steps. Place your hands on your hips.

Pyramid Pose Parsvottanasana (PARZH-voh-tahn-AHS-uh-nuh)
Heels in a strait line, toes pointing toward the top of mat. Point your left toes at the top-left corner of your mat, turned about 60 degrees. In a "scissored" kind of stance. With the torso facing the same direction as your front foot, square your hips to the top of the mat, shoulder blades firmly into your back.
Inhale as you reach your arms out to the sides. As you exhale, reach your arms behind your back. Clasp each elbow with the opposite hand. If your shoulders are more flexible, bring your hands into reverse prayer position, pressing your palms together and reaching your fingers toward your head.
On an inhalation, elongate your torso. Exhaling, fold at the hips and extend your torso over your front leg. Keep your shoulders drawing back, maintaining length in the spine. Crown of the head extends forward and tailbone extending behind. Be sure to fold from the hip, not the waist.
Gaze at your front big toe.
Release to **Standing forward fold Forward Bend** Uttanasana
Vinyasa through
Plank Pose Kumbhakasana
Cobra Pose Bhujangasana (boo-jang-GAHS-uh-nah)
Downward Dog Adho Mukha Svanasana

Down Dog Split LEFT LEG Tri Pada Adho Mukha Svanasana Left leg extends towards the sky. Bring the left leg forward through the hands. Left knee at 90 degree angle and come up for **Warrior I** Virabhadrasana I (Veer-ah-bah-DRAHS-ana)
Arms strait up towards the sky. Create 1 long line of energy from your back heel through the tips of your fingers.
Interlace fingers behind you. **Devotional/Humble Warrior** Baddha Virabhadrasana (ba-DAH Veer-ah-bah-DRAHS-ana)
Inhale expanding chest and lungs. As you exhale, continue to keep your heart open and gently bow forward, while your arms extend backward and upward. The left shoulder may graze the left leg even further to the left as you release your pelvis and drop deeper into the pose.
As you come up, place blocks on the front corners of the top of mat on the tallest height, Move to **Warrior II** Virabhadrasana II
Arms out to a T, relax the shoulders down.
Glance to see your blocks are in place for **Half Moon Pose** Ardha Chandrasana (ARD-uh chan-DRAHS-uh-nuh)
Reach through your left hand. Shift your right hip back, and then fold sideways and forward at the hip. Rest your left hand's fingertips onto your block. Align your shoulders so your right shoulder is directly above your left shoulder.
Bring your right hand to rest on your right hip.
Straighten your left leg while simultaneously lifting your right leg. Work to bring the right leg parallel to the floor, or even higher than your hips.
Reach actively through your right heel. Take care to not lock the left leg's knee. Stack top hip directly over your bottom hip, and open your torso to the right.
Then extend your right arm and point your fingertips directly toward the sky.
Balance. Find a **drishti** point, or an unmoving point of focus.

Draw your shoulderblades firmly into your back. Lengthen your tailbone toward your right heel.
To release, lower your right leg as you exhale, and shift back to **Warrior II** Virabhadrasana II
Triangle Pose Utthita Trikonasana (oo-TEE-tah tree-koh-NAH-suh-nuh)
Keep the left foot out so your toes are pointing to the top of the mat, and straiten the front leg.

Your arms should be aligned directly over your legs. With your palms facing down, reach actively from fingertip to fingertip.
On an exhalation, reach through your left hand in the same direction as your left foot is pointed. Shift your right hip back and fold down at your left hip. Keep your left ear, shoulder, and knee on the same plane (as if you are tipping like a teapot or moving within 2 panes of glass) Reach up with the right arm, fingertips reaching toward the sky. Align your shoulders so your right shoulder is directly above your left shoulder. Move the block directly next to and behind the left heel. As you tip down, place your left hand's fingertips on the block.
Gaze up toward the sky.

Stand at the top of your mat **Mountain Pose** Tadasana
Place the LEFT leg back about 3 to 4. Place your hands on your hips.
Pyramid Pose Parsvottanasana (PARZH-voh-tahn-AHS-uh-nuh)
Heels in a strait line, toes pointing toward the top of mat. Point your right toes at the top-right corner of your mat, turned about 60 degrees. In a "scissored" kind of stance. With the torso facing the same direction as your front foot, square your hips to the top of the mat, shoulder blades firmly into your back.
Inhale as you reach your arms out to the sides. As you exhale, reach your arms behind your back. Clasp each elbow with the opposite hand. If your shoulders are more flexible, bring your hands into reverse prayer position, pressing your palms together and reaching your fingers toward your head.
On an inhalation, elongate your torso. Exhaling, fold at the hips and extend your torso over your front leg. Keep your shoulders drawing back, maintaining length in the spine. Crown of the head extends forward and tailbone extending behind. Be sure to fold from the hip, not the waist.
Gaze at your front big toe.
Release to **Standing Forward Bend** Uttanasana
Vinyasa through
Plank Pose Kumbhakasana
Cobra Pose Bhujangasana (boo-jang-GAHS-uh-nah)
Downward Dog Adho Mukha Svanasana

Now, place the blocks beneath the feet on their lowest height for
Downward Dog Adho Mukha Svanasana
This will deepen the posture and provide an interesting challenge.
Walk up to stand into **Mountain Pose** Tadasana
Stand on top of the blocks on lowest height.

Fold down, **Standing Forward Bend** Uttanasana **into Ragdoll** Uttanasana variation
Let upper body hang over the legs, grab opposite elbows, head and neck are free and hang long.
Step off the blocks and stand behind them.
Place 1 block at it's narrowest height between your thighs and sit into **Chair Pose** Utkatasana (OOT-kuh-TAHS-uh-nuh) Hands at heart center. Take a deep inhale.
Chair Pose Twist to the RIGHT Parivrtta Utkatasana (PAHR-ee-VREE-tah OOT-kuh-TAHS-uh-nuh)

Exhaling, twist your torso to the right. Bring your left elbow to the outside of your right thigh. Shift your left hip back slightly, squaring off your hips once again. Bring your knees into alignment.
To deepen the pose, extend both arms, reaching your right fingertips to the sky and your left fingertips to the mat. In this deepened variation, option to place the left fingertips on a block.
Back to center **Chair Pose** Utkatasana

Push to **Downward Dog** now choosing how you'd like to place the blocks, another variation is placing your head on a block.
Walk up to **Mountain Pose** Tadasana and stand on blocks.
Fold down, **Standing Forward Bend** Uttanasana **into Ragdoll** Uttanasana variation
Let upper body hang over the legs, grab opposite elbows, head and neck are free and hang long.
Place 1 block at it's narrowest height between your thighs and sit into **Chair Pose** Utkatasana Hands at heart center. Take a deep inhale.
Chair Pose Twist to the LEFT Parivrtta Utkatasana
Exhaling, twist your torso to the left. Bring your right elbow to the outside of your left thigh. Shift your right hip back slightly, squaring off your hips once again. Bring your knees into alignment.
To deepen the pose, extend both arms, reaching your left fingertips to the sky and your right fingertips to the mat. In this deepened variation, option to place the right fingertips on a block.
Back to center **Chair Pose** Utkatasana
And back to **Downward Dog** Adho Mukha Svanasana

Table Pose Bharmanasana (Bar-man-AHS-un-nah)
Prepare for inversion:
Feathered Peacock Pose Pincha Mayurasana (pin-chah my-yur-AHS-anna)
Kneel on the floor. Clasp your elbows with opposite hands and place them on the ground in front of you.
Keep your elbows where they are, but release your hands and bring them forward so your forearms are parallel to one another, palms facing down.
Curl your toes under and straighten your legs. Walk your feet toward you until your hips are over your shoulders.
Lift one leg to the sky. Then bend knees slightly and push off the floor to lift both legs toward the sky. Balance in the pose for several breaths.
When you are ready, exhale and carefully lower both feet to the floor.

Relax and sit in **Easy Pose** Sukhasana

Release the legs into **Staff Pose** Dandasana (dan-DAHS-ah-nah) sitting on a block on its shortest height.
Sit for **Cobbler's Pose/Bound Ankle Pose** Baddha Konasana (BAH-duh cone-AHS-uh-nuh) sitting on a block.
Soles of the feet together, let knees drop to both sides. Clasp big toes with thumb and first finger. Extend the length of your entire spine skyward. Hold for 5 counts of breath. Fold Forward with a flat back. Pause for 5-7 breaths

Transition to lay on the back for a **Psoas Stretch:**
Our psoas muscle is the longest muscle in our body.

Hug the knees into the chest and create a circular motion with the back.
Circle one way, and then the other.
Hug the right knee into the armpit.
Let the left leg extend long and feel the stretch in the psoas muscle.
Bring the right knee over the body to the left side for a twist
Bring both knees into chest again.
Hug the left knee into armpit
Let the right leg extend long and feel the stretch in the psoas muscle.
Bring the left knee over the body to the right side for a twist.
Bring both knees into chest again.

Supported Fish Pose Matsyasana (maht-see-AHS-uh-nuh) is a great back-bending heart opener.
Place one yoga block vertically on the middle height where you think your shoulder blades will rest when you lie back and place another yoga block horizontally on the shortest height where you think your head will rest comfortably.
Gently release your back onto the shoulder block so that your shoulder blades are just above the block (the block will be at your middle back just grazing the bottom of your shoulder blades). Then, release your head to the second block so that it is comfortable for your neck, adjusting the block heights as needed. Allow your arms to relax on either side of you, and breathe here for at least five deep breaths.
If the back bend is too intense with the shoulder block on the middle height, lower it to the shortest height. Sink into the posture.
Allow gravity to sink the body so the heart opens.

Set the blocks off to the side and extend into **Relaxation Pose** Savasana (sha-VAHS-ah-nuh)
Moving onto the back. Allow legs to fall open. Eyes closed and relaxed.
Soften your face. Part lips slightly.

Closing Meditation
golden light yoga nidra
(Guided Savasana)

Bring your awareness to your breathing.
I will ask you to move your mind to different parts of your relaxed body.
When your mind moves to each part, imagine that part is being touched with a golden light.
There's no need to move that part of your body; simply move your imagination and that golden light there. We will move from relaxed part to relaxed part, lighting each part with golden light.
Begin with your left-hand thumb, index finger, third finger, ring finger, pinky, palm, wrist, forearm, elbow, shoulder, all filled with golden light.
Move to the right-hand thumb, index finger, third finger, ring finger, pinky, palm, wrist, forearm, elbow, shoulder, all filled with golden light.
Move down to the left big toe, second toe, third toe, fourth toe, pinky toe, top of foot, ankle, knee, thigh, hip. Golden light.
Then over to the right big toe, second toe, third toe, fourth toe, pinky toe, top of foot, ankle, knee, thigh, hip, all filled with golden light.
Move the light to your lower back, your upper back, neck, head, top of head, right ear, left ear, right eyebrow, left eyebrow, right eye, left eye, nose tip, upper lip, lower lip, jaw, tongue, throat, all filled with golden light. Then down to your chest, belly, heart, all filled with golden light."

Expanding the Light:
Now use you power within and share the wonderful light in your hearts. Think of all the people in the world that you love, and imagine sending them the golden light that you have pouring out through your heart. Your relatives, your sister, your brother, mother, father, your best friends, all your friends, your boss, your teachers, everyone you know. Now think of all the people in the world who could use some extra light in their lives, Maybe include someone that challenges you... and send the light it to them.
Now imagine all of these individuals returning this light back to you while you send it to them.

Come to a comfortable seated posture.
Closing with Breath: Breathe into your belly and feel that light moving out and coming in. Feel your belly ballooning out and in.
You are wonderful, special, unique, and the world needs your light.
Hands at heart center. Namaste.

Move Chill Yoga
Portable Yoga Class Plan 5
power within

Easy Pose
Table Pose
Extended Puppy Pose
Hero Pose
Downward Dog
Standing Forward Bend
Mountain Pose
Standing Forward Bend

High Lunge RIGHT leg back	High Lunge LEFT leg back
High Plank	High Plank
Side Plank	Side Plank
Wild Thing variation	Wild Thing variation
High Plank	High Plank
Chaturanga	Chaturanga
Upward Dog	Upward Dog
Downward Dog	Downward Dog

Standing Forward Bend
Mountain Pose

Downward Dog Split RIGHT LEG	Downward Dog Split LEFT LEG
Warrior I	Warrior I
Devotional Warrior	Devotional Warrior
Warriror II	Warrior II
Half Moon Pose	Half Moon Pose
Warrior II	Warrior II
Triangle Pose	Triangle Pose
Mountain Pose	Mountain Pose
Pyramid Pose	Pyramid Pose
Standing Forward Bend	Standing Forward Bend
Plank Pose	Plank Pose
Cobra Pose	Cobra Pose
Downward Dog	Downward Dog

Mountain Pose	Mountain Pose
Standing Forward Bend / Ragdoll	Standing Forward Bend / Ragdoll
Chair Pose	Chair Pose
Chair Pose Twist RIGHT	Chair Pose Twist LEFT
Downward Dog	Downward Dog

Table Pose
Inversion – Feathered Peacock Pose
Easy Pose
Staff Pose
Cobbler's Pose
Psoas stretches RIGHT and LEFT
Supported Fish Pose
Relaxation Pose

breath is life

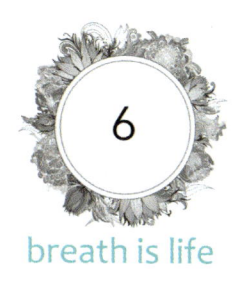

Opening Meditation
pranayama

We charge our cells phones every night, but how do you recharge your mind? We can do this through Pranayama.

Pranayamas are yogic breathing exercises that have the ability to quickly increase our energy, release stress, improve our mental clarity, and improve our physical health. Pranayama goes a step further than simple awareness of the breath, using specific rhythms and techniques to bring us numerous benefits on the mental, emotional and physical levels. It calms the mind, reduces worries and anxieties, improves focus and attention, removes brain fog, increases energy, brings enthusiasm and positivity, boosts the immune system, rejuvenates the body and mind, and may even slow down the aging process

Connections between breath and emotion:
Our breath is linked to our emotions. For every emotion, there is a particular rhythm in the breathing. When we experience anger or worry, we breathe faster. When we are calm and relaxed, we breathe slowly and comfortably.

If we understand the rhythm of our breath, we are able to control what is happening in the mind. We can ease negative impulses and emotions like anger, jealousy, greed, and we are able to live happier healthier lives.

> Place your hand on the belly. Close your eyes. Try your best to relax the rest of your body.
> On the Exhale, squeeze belly towards spine
> Inhale belly comes forward
> On the Exhale, squeeze belly towards spine
> Inhale belly comes forward
> On the Exhale, squeeze belly towards spine
> Do a couple more at your own pace.
> Place other hand on lower back. You can breathe with your back as well.
> Imagine you are expanding backwards also.
> Inhale expanding belly out and expanding spine outward towards the back body.
> Exhale squeezing belly in towards your spine
> Inhale expanding front and back   Exhale squeeze.
> Inhale expand   Exhale squeeze
> Inhale expand   Exhale squeeze

Open your eyes and notice how you feel after practicing deliberate breathing. We can come back to this practice and control our breath whenever we feel unease.

Begin in **Crocodile Pose** Makarasana (mah-kar-AHS-uh-nuh)
Stretch out on the mat face down. Extended legs a little wider then hip distance apart. Toes turned out, heels turned in. Fold your arms and place your hands on opposite elbows. Shoulders and head are off the mat. Rest the forehead on the forearms. Close the eyes and relax the body. This is a perfect posture for diaphragmatic breathing. The abdomen is isolated, as it is gently pressed to the floor.
Stay in Crocodile Pose Makarasana for 5-7 breath counts.

Bring your legs in for **Child's Pose** Balasana (bah-LAHS-ah-nuh)
Extend arms out, melt heart down, place forehead to mat, knees wide apart.
Pause again for 5-7 breath counts.

Come to **Table Pose** Bharmanasana (bar-ma-NAHS-ah-nah)
Create a flow through **Cow Pose** Bitilasana (bee-tee-LAHS-uh-nuh) and **Cat Pose** Marjaryasana (mahr-jahr-ee-AHS-uh-nuh)
Cow Pose: Inhale as you drop the belly towards the mat. Lift the chin and chest, and gaze up toward the ceiling. Broaden across your shoulder blades and draw your shoulders away from your ears.
Cat Pose: As you exhale, draw your belly to the spine and round the back toward the ceiling. Release the crown of your head toward the floor. Inhale, coming back into Cow Pose, and then exhale as you return to Cat Pose. Repeat 5-10 times, and then rest by sitting back on your heels with your torso upright.
Stand in **Mountain Pose** Tadasana (Ta-DAHS-un-nah) for a Sun Salutation

Sun Salutation using Cow Pose and Cat Pose
- Mountain Tadasana
- Standing Forward Bend Uttanasana (OO-tan-AHS-un-nah)
- Lunge Right leg back Anjaneyasana (AHN-jah-nay-AHS-uh-nuh)
- Downward Dog Adho Mukha Svanasana (AH-doh MOO-kah-shvah-Nahs-ana)
- Cow Bitilasana
- Cat Marjaryasana
- Downward Dog Adho Mukha Svanasana
- Lunge Left leg back Anjaneyasana
- Downward Dog Adho Mukha Svanasana
- Cow Bitilasana
- Cat Marjaryasana
- Downward Dog Adho Mukha Svanasana
- Standing Forward Bend Uttanasana
- Mountain Tadasana

X 3

Come to **Hero Pose** Vajrasana (vahj-RAHS-uh-nuh)
Kneeling on the floor, sit on the heels. Inhale arms all the way up. Bring hands down to heart center.

Gate Pose RIGHT Parighasana (par-ee-GOSS-anna)
Stretch your right leg out to the right and press the foot to the floor. Keep your left knee directly below your left hip (so the thigh is perpendicular to the floor), and align your right heel with the left knee. Point the kneecap toward the ceiling, which will require you to turn your right leg out. Bring your arms out to your sides, parallel to the floor, palms down. Bend to the right over the plane of the right leg and connect the right hand down on the shin, ankle, or the floor outside the right leg. Contract the right side of the torso and stretch the left. Place your left hand on the outer left hip. Create space in the left side.

Release and move to **Downward Dog** Adho Mukha Svanasana
Lift the hips, let your neck be soft. Press through all 10 fingers.

Low Lunge Anjaneyasana (AHN-jah-nay-AHS-uh-nuh)
RIGHT leg comes forward between hands. Frame the right foot with the hands. Extend the right arm skyward, keeping the left hand on the mat for **Revolved Lunge** to the right Parivrtta Anjaneyasana (PAHR-ee-VREE-tah AHN-jah-nay-AHS-uh-nuh)

Back to **Downward Dog** Adho Mukha Svanasana

Come to **Hero Pose** Vajrasana (vahj-RAHS-uh-nuh)
Kneeling on the floor, sit on the heels. Inhale arms all the way up. Bring hands down to heart center.

Gate Pose LEFT Parighasana (par-ee-GOSS-anna)
Stretch your left leg out to the left and press the foot to the floor. Keep your right knee directly below your right hip (so the thigh is perpendicular to the floor), and align your left heel with the right knee. Point the kneecap toward the ceiling, which will require you to turn your left leg out. Bring your arms out to your sides, parallel to the floor, palms down. Bend to the left over the plane of the left leg and connect the left hand down on the shin, ankle, or the floor outside the left leg. Contract the left side of the torso and stretch the right. Place your right hand on the outer right hip. Create space in the right side.

Release and move to **Downward Dog** Adho Mukha Svanasana
(Lift the hips, let your neck be soft. Press through all 10 fingers.

Low Lunge Anjaneyasana
LEFT leg comes forward between hands. Frame the left foot with the hands. Extend the left arm skyward, keeping the right hand on the mat for **Revolved Lunge** to the left Parivrtta Anjaneyasana

Back to **Downward Dog** Adho Mukha Svanasana

Walk up to **Mountain Pose** Tadasana
Warrior I Virabhadrasana I (Veer-ah-bah-DRAHS-ana) – open RIGHT leg back
Extend arms out to a T into **Warrior II** Virabhadrasana II Gaze is forward. Shoulders down and relaxed. Breathe.

Bring arms to **Cow Face arms** Gomukhasana (go-moo-KAHS-uh-nuh)
Extend your left arm up toward the ceiling with your palm facing forward. Then, bend your left elbow and bring your left hand to your spine, beneath the neck. Extend your right arm to the side with your palm facing down. Internally rotate your arm so your palm faces behind you. Then, bend your right elbow and bring

your right hand up the center of your back. Tuck your forearm into the hollow of your low back.
Roll your shoulders back and down. If possible, hook the fingers of both hands. Reach your top elbow toward the ceiling while reaching your lower elbow toward the floor. Broaden across your collar bones. Gaze gently upward. Keep your eyes and breath relaxed. Lengthen through the crown of your head.

Stand in **Mountain Pose** Tadasana

King Dancer Pose Natarajasana (NOT-ah-rahj-AHS-uh-nuh) RIGHT leg
Bring your right heel toward your right buttock. Reach your right hand down and clasp your right foot's inner ankle. You can also loop a strap around the top of your right foot, and then hold onto the strap with your right hand. Reach your left arm overhead, pointing your fingertips toward the ceiling and facing your palm to the right. Fix your gaze softly at a **drishti** point or unmoving point of focus. Make sure your left kneecap and toes point directly forward.
When you feel steady, begin to lift your right foot away from your body as you lean your torso slightly forward. Keep your chest lifted and continue reaching your left hand's fingertips up toward the ceiling. Raise your right foot as high as you can.

Compress down into **Goddess Pose** Utkata Konasana (oot-KAH-tuh cone-AHS-uh-nuh)
Step your feet wide apart. Turn your toes out slightly, so they point to the corners of your mat. Exhale, bend your knees directly over your toes and lower your hips into a squat. Work toward bringing your thighs parallel to the floor. Extend your arms out to the sides with your palms facing down. Bend your elbows and point your fingertips toward the ceiling; your upper arms and forearms should be at a 90-degree angle, also known as "Cactus arms".
Tuck your tailbone in slightly and press your hips forward as you draw your thighs back. Keep your knees in line with your toes. Soften your shoulders. Gaze softly at the horizon.
Hold for up to 10 breaths.

Mountain Pose Tadasana
Warrior I Virabhadrasana I – open LEFT leg back
Extend arms out to a T into **Warrior II** Virabhadrasana II Gaze is forward. Shoulders down and relaxed. Breathe.
Bring arms to **Cow Face arms** Gomukhasana
Extend your right arm up toward the ceiling with your palm facing forward. Then, bend your right elbow and bring your right hand to your spine, beneath the neck. Extend your left arm to the side with your palm facing down. Internally rotate your arm so your palm faces behind you. Then, bend your left elbow and bring your left hand up the center of your back. Tuck your forearm into the hollow of your low back.
Roll your shoulders back and down. If possible, hook the fingers of both hands. Reach your top elbow toward the ceiling while reaching your lower elbow toward the floor. Broaden across your collar bones. Gaze gently upward. Keep your eyes and breath relaxed. Lengthen through the crown of your head.

Stand in **Mountain Pose** Tadasana

King Dancer Pose Natarajasana LEFT leg
Bring your left heel toward your left buttock. Reach your left hand down and clasp your left foot's inner ankle. You can also loop a strap around the top of your left foot, and then hold onto the strap with your left hand. Reach your right arm overhead, pointing your fingertips toward the ceiling and facing your palm to the left. Fix your gaze softly at a **drishti** point or unmoving point of focus. Make sure your right kneecap and toes point directly forward.
When you feel steady, begin to lift your left foot away from your body as you lean your torso slightly forward. Keep your chest lifted and continue reaching your right hand's fingertips up toward the ceiling. Raise your left foot as high as you can

Compress again into **Goddess Pose** Utkata Konasana
Hold for up to 10 breaths.

Push to **Downward Dog** Adho Mukha Svanasana
Lift head up and slowly shift the weight of the body to the front placing hands and forearms flat on the mat. Elbows beneath shoulders into **Dolphin Pose** Makarasana (makar-AHS-uh-nuh)
Lower the legs down for **Sphinx Pose** Salamba Bhujangasana (sah-LOM-bah boo-jahn-GAHS-uh-nuh) keeping the forearms flat on the mat. Lift the head and chest, press pubic bone to the mat and strongly engage the legs.

Half Frog Pose Ardha Bhekasana (ar-duh Be-KAHS-ah-nah)
Come up onto your RIGHT fingertips. Bend your right knee and draw your right heel in toward your seat. Catch hold of the big-toe side of your foot with your right hand, bending your elbow to draw your heel in toward you for the thigh stretch. Continue to lift up through your low belly, and keep your rib cage and chest facing forward. Remain in the pose for a few breaths. Release on an exhale.
Repeat **Half Frog Pose** Ardha Bhekasana with LEFT
Come up onto your LEFT fingertips. Bend your left knee and draw your left heel in toward your seat. Catch hold of the big-toe side of your foot with your left hand, bending your elbow to draw your heel in toward you for the thigh stretch. Continue to lift up through your low belly, and keep your rib cage and chest facing forward.
Remain in the pose for a few breaths. Release on an exhale.

Downward Dog Adho Mukha Svanasana
Down Dog Split RIGHT LEG Tri Pada Adho Mukha Svanasana
Right leg extends towards the sky. Bring the right shin forward through the hands for
One-Leg King Pigeon Pose varitation RIGHT Eka Pada Raja Kapotasana
(aa-KAH pah-DAH rah-JAH-cop-poh-TAHS-anna)
With right knee near the right wrist, press the pinky-toe side of your foot into the floor so that your heel lifts up and your front ankle stays straight.
To set up for the thigh stretch, draw your left heel in toward your seat and catch hold of the big-toe side of your foot with your left hand. Square your rib cage and chest toward the front of the mat.

Downward Dog Adho Mukha Svanasana
Down Dog Split LEFT LEG Tri Pada Adho Mukha Svanasana
Left leg extends towards the sky. Bring the left shin forward through the hands for
One-Leg King Pigeon Pose varitation LEFT Eka Pada Raja Kapotasana
With left knee near the left wrist, press the pinky-toe side of your foot into the floor so that your heel lifts up and your front ankle stays straight.
To set up for the thigh stretch, draw your right heel in toward your seat and catch hold of the big-toe side of your foot with your left hand. Square your rib cage and chest toward the front of the mat.

Release again to **Downward Dog** Adho Mukha Svanasana
Deep breath - All 10 fingers and palms pressing into mat, hips up as if a string is pulling up the hips, gaze at belly button
Find stillness.
Walk the feet in and move to a **Wide Leg Forward Bend** Prasarita Padottanasana (prah-suh-REE-tuh pah-doh-tahn-AHS-uh-nuh) – Arms come out
Twist to the right, Bending down with a flat back, bringing the left hand to the right shin or foot, wherever it is comfortable. Keeping arms wide, switch to touch the left shin or foot with the right hand. Look towards the sky with each side change. Continue to Windmill the arms here while coordinating the breath.

Stand in **Mountain Pose** Tadasana

Eagle Pose Garudasana (gahr-ooo-DAHS-uh-nuh)
Bend your knees. Balance on your RIGHT foot and cross your left thigh over your right. Fix your gaze at a point in front of you. Hook the top of your left foot behind your right calf. Balance for one breath.
(Omit the foot hook and cross the leg over the top of the standing leg, for a less intense variation)
Extend your arms straight in front of your body. Move your left arm under your right. Bend your elbows, and then raise your forearms perpendicular to the floor. Wrap your hands, and press your palms together (or as close as you can get them). Lift your elbows and reach your fingertips toward the ceiling. Keep your shoulder blades pressing down your back, toward your waist.
Square your hips. Breathe smoothly and evenly.
Hold for up to one minute, focusing on your breath and keeping your gaze fixed and soft. Gently unwind your arms and legs.
Move back into **Mountain Pose** Tadasana
Repeat **Eagle Pose** Garudasana on the other side.
Bend your knees. Balance on your LEFT foot and cross your right thigh over your left. Fix your gaze at a point in front of you. Hook the top of your right foot behind your left calf. Balance for one breath.
(Omit the foot hook and cross the leg over the top of the standing leg, for a less intense variation)
Extend your arms straight in front of your body. Move your right arm under your left. Bend your elbows, and then raise your forearms perpendicular to the floor.
Wrap your hands, and press your palms together (or as close as you can get them).

Lift your elbows and reach your fingertips toward the ceiling. Keep your shoulder blades pressing down your back, toward your waist.
Square your hips. Breathe smoothly and evenly.
Hold for up to one minute, focusing on your breath and keeping your gaze fixed and soft. Gently unwind your arms and legs
Move back into **Mountain Pose** Tadasana

Lay flat on the mat face down, returning to **Crocodile Pose** Makarasana
Extended legs a little wider then hip distance apart. Toes turned out, heels turned in.
Fold your arms and place your hands on opposite elbows. Shoulders and head are off the mat. Rest the forehead on the forearms.
Close the eyes and relax the body. Relax for several breath counts.
Prepare for a back bend.

Bow Pose Dhanurasana (DAHN-yoor-AHS-uh-nuh)
On an exhalation, bend knees. Bring your heels as close as you can to your buttocks, keeping your knees hip-distance apart. Reach back with both hands and hold onto your outer ankles.
Lift the heels up toward the ceiling, drawing your thighs up and off the mat. Your head, chest, and upper torso will also lift off the mat. Lift your chest and press your shoulder blades firmly into your upper back. Draw your shoulders away from your ears. Your breath may become shallow, but do not hold your breath.
Hold for up to 30 seconds.
Release and lower your thighs to the mat. Slowly release your legs and feet to the floor. Repeat the pose x 2, for the same amount of time.

Come to **Table Pose** Bharmanasana and prepare for handstand by pressing the soles of your feet onto a wall.
L-Pose Handstand Adho Mukha Vrksasana(ah-doh moo-kah vriks-SHAHS-anna)
Tuck your toes under on the floor and straighten your legs. With heels on the wall, come into a shortened version of Down Dog at the wall. It might feel like you are too close to the wall, but that's ok. Press the palms down into the mat and your arms straight as you take one foot up the wall with your toes curled under at about the height of your hips. Begin to straighten the raised leg, pressing the sole of your foot into the wall, and sending your hips over your shoulders as you bring the second leg up to join the first.

Release down and come to lie on the back for **Reclined Goddess**
Supta Baddha Konasana (SOOP-tah BAH-duh cone-AHS-uh-nuh)
Bring your elbows to the floor and the soles of the feet together, knees open to the sides. Adjust your position so your spine lengthens along the floor while maintaining the natural curve of the lower back. Draw your shoulder blades inward, let your arms relax with your palms facing up. Lengthen your tailbone toward your heels. Close your eyes and bring your awareness to your breath.
Allow your body to feel heavy for 10 counts of breath.

Come up to a seat in **Easy Pose** Sukhasana for **Yoga Mudra** – yoga seal (seal of the practice) Close the eyes and take a few easy breaths. Try to reflect upon the experience of the asana session, on the extra energy (prana) generated in the system.
Clasp the elbows behind the back. Take a deep breath in and while exhaling slowly, begin to bend forward. Try to bend at with a flat back from the waist. Bring the forehead down as far as comfortable.
Stay in the final pose for about 6-7 breaths.

Come up and lay all the way back for **Relaxation Pose** Savasana (sha-VAHS-ah-nuh)
Moving onto the back. Allow legs to fall open. Eyes closed and relaxed.
Soften your face. Part lips slightly.

Closing Meditation
intention from the core

Sit tall in **Easy Pose** Sukhasana, or any comfortable position
Feel relaxation in your face and eyes
Allow the chest to expand as you inhale
As you exhale, fully relax the shoulders away from the ears

Place a hand on your abdomen
Fill up your entire core with breath as you inhale
Release the breath from your core as you exhale

Allow the warm breath to burn away any unnecessary tension,
negative emotion, and stress.
Instead, the warm air strengthens and empowers you
On an inhale, visualize breathing in a spiral of flames
in bright fiery warm colors and golden light.
The fire fuels you with happiness, health, success, and energy.

Next, decide how you would like to feel right now
Choose a feeling that feels right to you
Now, with each breath, say that feeling and feel that feeling in your core

Breathe in your intention, Breathe out your intention

Some examples are, if you'd like to feel confidence today
Breathe in confidence, Breathe out confidence

If you want to feel motivated today
Breathe in motivation, Breathe out motivation

Let your breath bring the feeling to your core.
Now, let the feeling expand throughout the body.

Continue with the breath for a few more rounds, expanding the feeling even further.

Move Chill Yoga
Portable Yoga Class Plan 6
breath is life

Crocodile Pose
Child's Pose
Table Pose
Cow and Cat
Sun Salutation with Cow and Cat x 3
- Mountain Pose
- Standing Forward Bend
- Lunge Right leg back
- Downward Dog
- Cow Pose
- Cat Pose
- Downward Dog
- Lunge Left leg back
- Downward Dog
- Cow Pose
- Cat Pose
- Downward Dog
- Standing Forward Bend
- Mountain Pose

X 3

Hero Pose	**Hero Pose**
Gate Pose RIGHT	**Gate Pose LEFT**
Downward Dog	**Downward Dog**
Low Lunge RIGHT leg forward	**Low Lunge LEFT leg forward**
Revolved Lunge	**Revolved Lunge**
Downward Dog	**Downward Dog**
Mountain Pose	**Mountain Pose**
Warrior I	**Warrior I**
Warrior II	**Warrior II**
Cow Face arms	**Cow Face arms**
Mountain Pose	**Mountain Pose**
King Dancer Pose RIGHT leg back	**King Dancer Pose LEFT leg back**
Goddess Pose	**Goddess Pose**

Downward Dog
Dolphin Pose
Sphinx Pose
Half Frog Pose Right and Left

Downward Dog Split RIGHT leg	**Downward Dog Split LEFT leg**
One-Leg King Pigeon Pose	**One-Leg King Pigeon Pose**
Downward Dog	**Downward Dog**

Wide Leg Forward Bend / Windmill arms
Mountain Pose
Eagle Pose Winding arms and legs RIGHT then LEFT
Mountain Pose
Crocodile Pose
Bow Pose
Table Pose
L-Shape Handstand
Reclined Goddess
Easy Pose / Yoga Mudra
Relaxation Pose

7

colder seasons

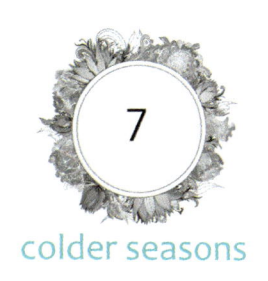

Opening Meditation
grounding

Cold air produces dryness and changes outside, but also changes in us.
We start to have symptoms such as lack of circulation, dry skin, and dehydration.
We have more air and space active in our bodies.
Tension collects, which can lead to restlessness and anxious thoughts.
Be sure to stay hydrated and consume more citrus, root veggies, cinnamon, and winter greens such as brussel sprouts.
This is a practice that focuses on replenishing our bodies to prepare for colder seasons.

Sit in a comfortable seated position such as **Hero Pose** Virasana (veer-AHS-un-nuh)
Close your eyes
Imagine an old tree, rooted deep underground
Imagine the life force in its roots
Imagine the size, the tree bark, its texture, branches, leaves
The breeze blowing through it
See the beauty of the leaves softly falling with ease on a soft white frost in the grass
See the feeling of the cold weather season reflected in the tree

Now, broaden the vision out to many trees, or a forest
See the forest as if you are floating above and looking down
From here, really see all the changes happening in nature.
The treetops, the sea of leaves below them on the ground, the colors of the trees and leaves

Move your vision back to the trunk and root of the single tree

Now, bring the vision to yourself and how it feels to be rooted and grounded

Bring your attention to the breath: Feel present. Our bodies tend to rush.
On each inhalation, bring in energy.
Feel your heart beating. Feel the energy in your heart. Slowly open your eyes

Easy Pose Twist Parivrtta Sukhasana (PAH-ruh-VREE-tah soo-KAHS-uh-nuh)
Balance your weight evenly across your sit bones. Relax your neck, shoulders, feet and thighs. Place your right hand on the floor behind you. Bring your left hand to the outside of your right knee, gently twisting to the right. Inhale to lengthen your spine, and exhale to twist deeper. Gaze over your right shoulder.
Hold for 5-7 breath counts.
Come back to center. Change the cross of your legs.
Place your left hand on the floor behind you. Bring your right hand to the outside of your left knee, gently twisting to the left. Inhale to lengthen your spine, and exhale to twist deeper. Gaze over your left shoulder. 5-7 breath counts.
Come up to stand in **Mountain Pose** Tadasana (Ta-DAHS-un-nah)

Sun Salutation B Surya Namaskara
With Sun Salutation B, practice breathing through the nose, which warms the air, just as the **vinyasa** warms up the body. Vin-YAHS-ah - **movement/flowing sequence in coordination with the breath**. Exhale when bending or folding and inhale when extending.
- Mountain pose Tadasana
- Chair pose Utkatasana (OOT-kuh-TAHS-uh-nuh)
- Standing forward fold Uttanasana (OO-tan-AHS-un-nah)
- Half standing forward fold (coming up half way)
- Plank pose Kumbhakasana (koom-bahk-AHS-uh-nuh)
- Upward dog pose Urdhva Mukha Svanasana (ORD-vah MOO-kah shvon-AHS-anna)
- Downward dog pose Adho Mukha Svanasana (AH-doh MOO-kah-shvah-Nahs-ana)
- Warrior I (right leg back) Virabhadrasana I (Veer-ah-bah-DRAHS-ana)
- Low plank pose Kumbhakasana
- Upward dog pose Urdhva Mukha Svanasana
- Downward dog pose Adho Mukha Svanasana
- Warrior I (left leg back) Virabhadrasana I
- Low plank pose Kumbhakasana
- Upward dog pose Urdhva Mukha Svanasana
- Downward dog pose Adho Mukha Svanasana
- Half standing forward fold (coming up half way)
- Forward fold Uttanasana
- Chair pose Utkatasana
- Mountain pose Tadasana

Repeat X 3

Move to lay on the back and hug knees into chest.
Pause here and create little circles with the back. Revolve one way and then the other way.
Keeping the knees hugged in, move to lay on your RIGHT side for
Revolved Reclined Dancer Natarajasana variation (NOT-ah-rahj-AHS-uh-nuh)
Bring the left heel toward your left buttock. Reach your left arm to meet and hold the left foot. Keep the right arm flat on the mat with the palm facing up. Right knee is still bent, laying flat on the mat below the right arm. Raise the left leg skyward for the stretch and ease into a gentle reclined back bend for the left side.
Release and hug the knees back into the chest.

Keeping the knees hugged in, move to lay on your LEFT side for **Revolved Reclined Dancer** Natarajasana variation

Bring the right heel toward your right buttock. Reach your right arm to meet and hold the right foot. Keep the left arm flat on the mat with the palm facing up. Left knee is still bent, laying flat on the mat below the left arm. Raise the right leg skyward for the stretch and ease into a gentle reclined back bend for the right side. Release and hug both knees into chest.

Windshield wiper the legs back and forth, dropping the knees to the right and to the left.

Come to a seated position, **Firelog Pose** Agnistambhasana (AG-nee-stahm-BAHS-uh-nuh)
Bring your right ankle to rest just above your left kneecap. Bend your left knee. Slide your left shin beneath your right shin, bringing your left ankle directly underneath your right knee.

Work toward bringing your shins parallel to the top edge of your mat, keeping your right shin stacked directly above your left shin. Flex your feet and press through your heels. Spread your toes.

Sit up tall through the crown of your head. Rest your fingertips on the floor at either side of your body. Those who are more flexible can walk their hands forward along the floor, folding their torso over their crossed legs.

Hold for 5-7 counts of breath.

Release the pose by very slowly and gently extending both legs along the floor into **Staff Pose** Dandasana (dan-DAHS-ah-nah) legs extended out in front of you.

Flex your feet and press out through your heels. Keep your big toes, inner heels, and inner knees together. Engage your thigh muscles and stretch your heels away from your body

Repeat **Firelog Pose** Agnistambhasana for the same amount of time with the opposite leg on top.

Release again to **Staff Pose** Dandasana

Come to **Table Pose** Bharmanasana (Bar-man-AHS-un-nah)
Push to **Downward Dog** Adho Mukha Svanasana
Deep breath - All 10 fingers and palms pressing into mat, hips up as if a string is pulling up the hips, gaze at belly button
Find stillness
Move the RIGHT foot between hands **Low Lunge** Anjaneyasana (AHN-jah-nay-AHS-uh-nuh)
Arms strait overhead, rest on the ball of the left foot with the knee down. Then place the hands beside the right foot and straiten the right knee, moving the pelvis back slightly for a **Hamstring Stretch**
Come up to **Mountain Pose** Tadasana (Ta-DAHS-un-nah), raise arms up overhead and release down into **Standing Forward Bend** Uttanasana (OO-tan-AHS-un-nah)
Push back to **Downward Dog** Adho Mukha Svanasana
Move the LEFT foot between hands **Low Lunge** Anjaneyasana
Arms strait overhead, rest on the ball of the right foot with the knee down. Then place the hands beside the left foot and straiten the left knee, moving the pelvis back slightly for a **Hamstring Stretch**
Come up to **Mountain Pose** Tadasana raise arms up overhead and release down into **Standing Forward Bend** Uttanasana

Push to **Downward Dog** Adho Mukha Svanasana
Deep breath - All 10 fingers and palms pressing into mat, hips up as if a string is pulling up the hips, gaze at belly button
Find stillness

Stand in **Mountain Pose** Tadasana
Find balance in **Tree pose** Vrksasana (vrik-SHAH-suh-nuh) with the RIGHT leg lifted and the left leg grounded into the mat. Arms up and out, find a **drishti** point to focus your gaze and help with balance.
Tree Pose Twist toward the right side of the space, set your gaze to the right. Return to center.
Tree Pose Bend to the right. Bending from the waist, gently fold the body down to the right, feeling the stretch in the left side waist.
Stand back in **Mountain Pose** Tadasana
Find balance in **Tree pose** Vrksasana (vrik-SHAH-suh-nuh) with the LEFT leg lifted and the right leg grounded into the mat. Arms up and out, find a **drishti** point to focus your gaze and help with balance.
Tree Pose Twist toward the left side of the space, set your gaze to the left. Return to center.
Tree Pose Bend to the left. Bending from the waist, gently fold the body down to the left, feeling the stretch in the right side waist.

Back to **Mountain Pose** Tadasana Inhale.
Exhale **Standing Forward Bend** Uttanasana
Bending over legs with a flat back.

Move to **High Lunge** Anjaneyasana (AHN-jah-nay-AHS-uh-nuh) RIGHT leg back. Left knee bent at a 90 degree angle. Rest on the ball of the right foot. Arms overhead, reaching through the upper body. Move hands to heart center, palms together.
Twist the body to the left, press your upper right arm against your left thigh and revolve your chest to the left for **Crescent Lunge Twist** Parivrtta Anjaneyasana (PAHR-ee-VREE-tah AHN-jah-nay-AHS-uh-nuh)
Release hands to the floor to frame the front foot. Allow your right heel to come to the mat and raise arms into **Warrior I** Virabhadrasana I
Left knee is bent directly over the ankle so that the thigh is parallel to the floor. Bring arms up toward the ceiling. Chest stays open as you come into a slight backbend. Touch palms overhead or keep arms parallel pointing upward. Hips pointing forward.
Extend arms out to a T into **Warrior II** Virabhadrasana II Gaze is forward. Shoulders down and relaxed. Breathe.

Release down to **Plank Pose** Kumbhakasana
Lower knees, chest, chin, for **Cobra Pose** Bhujangasana (boo-jang-GAHS-uh-nah)
Hug elbows in, Press down through tops of feet. Inhale gently lift head and chest, shoulders back, heart forward. Gaze to the floor or up to the sky.
Tuck toes and push back to **Downward Dog** Adho Mukha Svanasana (AH-doh MOO-kah-shvah-Nahs-ana)
Deep breath - All 10 fingers and palms pressing into mat, hips up as if a string is pulling up the hips, gaze at belly button
Find stillness
Walk feet up to **Forward fold** Uttanasana
Stand in **Mountain Pose** Tadasana

Move to **High Lunge** Anjaneyasana LEFT leg back. Right knee bent at a 90 degree angle. Rest on the ball of the left foot. Arms overhead, reaching through the upper body. Move hands to heart center, palms together.

Twist the body to the right, press your upper left arm against your right thigh and revolve your chest to the right for **Crescent Lunge Twist** Parivrtta Anjaneyasana
Release hands to the floor to frame the front foot. Allow your left heel to come to the mat and raise arms into **Warrior I** Virabhadrasana I
Right knee is bent directly over the ankle so that the thigh is parallel to the floor. Bring arms up toward the ceiling. Chest stays open as you come into a slight backbend. Touch palms overhead or keep arms parallel pointing upward. Hips pointing forward.
Extend arms out to a T into **Warrior II** Virabhadrasana II Gaze is forward. Shoulders down and relaxed. Breathe.

Release down to **Plank Pose** Kumbhakasana
Lower knees, chest, chin, for **Cobra Pose** Bhujangasana (boo-jang-GAHS-uh-nah)
Hug elbows in, Press down through tops of feet. Inhale gently lift head and chest, shoulders back, heart forward. Gaze to the floor or up to the sky.
Tuck toes and push back to **Downward Dog** Adho Mukha Svanasana (AH-doh MOO-kah-shvah-Nahs-ana)
Deep breath - All 10 fingers and palms pressing into mat, hips up as if a string is pulling up the hips, gaze at belly button
Find stillness
Walk feet up to **Forward fold** Uttanasana
Stand in **Mountain Pose** Tadasana

High Lunge Anjaneyasana RIGHT leg back. Left knee bent at a 90 degree angle. Rest on the ball of the left right. Arms out to a T.
High Lunge Twist toward the left thigh. Revolve the waist to where it feels comfortable. Come back to center
Allow your right heel to come to the mat and raise arms into **Warrior I** Virabhadrasana I
Chest stays open as you come into a slight backbend. Hips pointing forward.

Straiten the front leg. **Pyramid Pose** Parsvottanasana (PARZH-voh-tahn-AHS-uh-nuh)
Heels in a strait line, toes pointing toward the top of mat. Stand in a "scissored" kind of stance, feet about 3 steps apart. With the torso facing the same direction as your front foot, square your hips to the top of the mat, shoulder blades firmly into your back.
Inhale as you reach your arms out to the sides. As you exhale, reach your arms behind your back. Clasp each elbow with the opposite hand. If your shoulders are more flexible, bring your hands into reverse prayer position, pressing your palms together and reaching your fingers toward your head.
On an inhalation, elongate your torso. Exhaling, fold at the hips and extend your torso over your front leg. Keep your shoulders drawing back, maintaining length in the spine. Crown of the head extends forward and tailbone extending behind. Be sure to fold from the hip, not the waist.
Gaze at your front big toe.

Release down to **Plank Pose** Kumbhakasana
Lower knees, chest, chin, for **Cobra Pose** Bhujangasana (boo-jang-GAHS-uh-nah)
Hug elbows in, Press down through tops of feet. Inhale gently lift head and chest, shoulders back, heart forward. Gaze to the floor or up to the sky.

Tuck toes and push back to **Downward Dog** Adho Mukha Svanasana
Deep breath - All 10 fingers and palms pressing into mat, hips up as if a string is pulling up the hips, gaze at belly button
Find stillness
Walk feet up to **Forward fold** Uttanasana
Stand in **Mountain Pose** Tadasana

High Lunge Anjaneyasana LEFT leg back. Right knee bent at a 90 degree angle. Rest on the ball of the leftfoot. Arms out to a T.
High Lunge Twist toward the right thigh. Revolve the waist to where it feels comfortable. Come back to center.
Allow your left heel to come to the mat and raise arms into **Warrior I** Virabhadrasana I
Chest stays open as you come into a slight backbend. Hips pointing forward.

Straiten the right leg. **Pyramid Pose** Parsvottanasana (PARZH-voh-tahn-AHS-uh-nuh)
Heels in a strait line, toes pointing toward the top of mat. Stand in a "scissored" kind of stance, feet about 3 steps apart. With the torso facing the same direction as your front foot, square your hips to the top of the mat, shoulder blades firmly into your back.
Inhale as you reach your arms out to the sides. As you exhale, reach your arms behind your back. Clasp each elbow with the opposite hand. If your shoulders are more flexible, bring your hands into reverse prayer position, pressing your palms together and reaching your fingers toward your head.
On an inhalation, elongate your torso. Exhaling, fold at the hips and extend your torso over your front leg. Keep your shoulders drawing back, maintaining length in the spine. Crown of the head extends forward and tailbone extending behind. Be sure to fold from the hip, not the waist.
Gaze at your front big toe.

Release down to **Plank Pose** Kumbhakasana
Lower knees, chest, chin, for **Cobra Pose** Bhujangasana (boo-jang-GAHS-uh-nah)
Hug elbows in, Press down through tops of feet. Inhale gently lift head and chest, shoulders back, heart forward. Gaze to the floor or up to the sky.
Tuck toes and push back to **Downward Dog** Adho Mukha Svanasana
Deep breath - All 10 fingers and palms pressing into mat, hips up as if a string is pulling up the hips, gaze at belly button
Find stillness
Walk feet up to **Forward fold** Uttanasana
Stand in **Mountain Pose** Tadasana

Chair Pose Utkatasana (OOT-kuh-TAHS-uh-nuh) Heart forward, weight to your heels, arms all the way up. Bend knees as if you are sitting in a chair. *You can place a block at it's narrowest width between your knees to increase strength in the abdominals and inner thighs.
Move onto the balls of both feet for **Elevated Chair Pose** Utkatasana Balance and hold.

Flatten feet to the floor and slowly bend the knees and squat down,
Yogi Squat Malasana (Mah-LAHS-ah-nah) being careful not to let the knees extend forward beyond the alignment of the feet.

Squatting down as far as possible, wiggle the shoulders in between the knees, using the elbows to push back against the inner knees, keeping the hands at heart center with the back straight and feet flat to the floor.

Bring knees down to sit into **Hero Pose** Virasana Kneeling on the floor, sit on the heels. Inhale arms all the way up. Bring hands down to heart center.
Extend to stretch the right arm up and over towards the left side of the space.
Arms back to center
Extend to stretch the left arm up and over towards the right side of the space.

Push to **Downward Dog** Adho Mukha Svanasana
Lift head up and slowly shift the weight of the body to the front, placing hands and forearms flat on the mat. Elbows beneath shoulders into **Dolphin Pose** Makarasana (makar-AHS-uh-nuh)
Lower the legs down for **Sphinx Pose** Salamba Bhujangasana (sah-LOM-bah boo-jahn-GAHS-uh-nuh) keeping the forearms flat on the mat. Lift the head and chest, press the pubic bone to the mat and strongly engage the legs. Tops of the feet resting into the mat.

Come to lay down with the front of the body on the mat
Half Bow Pose Ardha Dhanurasana (Ar-duh DAHN-yoor-AHS-uh-nuh)
With the legs together or a few inches apart. Bring the chin to the floor. Arms bent and palms flat on the mat.
Bend the RIGHT knee and swim the left hand back around to hold onto the right heel or ankle. Inhale and kick the right foot into the arm to lift the right leg, head and chest off of the floor. Press down into the right arm and hand for support.
Breathe and hold for 5-7 breaths.
To release: slowly exhale and lower the leg, arm, head and chest down to the floor.
Repeat **Half Bow Pose** Ardha Dhanurasana on other side. Bend the LEFT knee and swim the right arm around to hold the right heel or ankle.

Bring knees up to sit into **Hero Pose** Virasana Kneeling on the floor, sit on the heels. Inhale arms all the way up. Bring hands down to heart center.
Once you feel comfortable, place the hands on the floor behind you.

Reclining Hero Pose Supta Virasana (SOOP-tah veer-AHS-uh-nuh)
Lean your weight into your hands, then lower your elbows and forearms to the floor. Allow your thigh bones to release deep into your hip sockets. Move the knees slightly apart, but not wider than the hips. Rest your arms at your sides. Draw your inner groin up and into your pelvis. Create length between your vertebrae, and broaden across your collarbones.
With practice, the pose becomes restful and you might stay in it for 5-10 minutes. Release and gently press back up to **Hero Pose** Virasana

Tuck your knees into the chest and lower the body down on the mat for
Reclined Butterfly Supta Bada Konasana (SOOP-tah BAH-duh cone-AHS-uh-nuh)
Press the soles of your feet together and let your knees drop open to both sides. Draw your shoulder blades gently inward and let your arms relax with your palms facing up. Relax your buttocks and lengthen your tailbone toward your heels. Close your eyes. Let your awareness become fully internal.

Gently lift the legs and flex the feet, turning the soles of the feet skyward for
Dead Bug Ananda Balasana variation (AH-nan-duh bah-LAHS-anna)
With knees bent, widen the knees. Raise your arms to point skyward so all 4 limbs are extended toward the sky. Keep the sacrum flat on the mat.

Lower the legs and arms for **Relaxation Pose** Savasana (sha-VAHS-ah-nuh)
Palms facing up. Eyes closed and relaxed.

Closing Meditation
warming the body and mind

Ujjayi Pranayama (ooh-JAH-yee prah-nah-YAH-mah)
"Victorious breath" or "The Ocean" breath slows the breath and makes an audible sound. This sound can be an excellent point of focus for yoga and mediation. The Uijayi breath also warms up the body, and cleanses and warms the nasal passages.

Put 1 hand in front of your face, Imagine your hand is a mirror
Inhale in and Exhale through the mouth as if you are fogging a mirror
Repeat
Now try it breathing only with the nose.
Make the sound in your throat on the exhale.
Repeat

Close the eyes.
Continue breathing only through the nose, allowing each inhale to draw in warmth.
Exhale anything you no longer need to hold on to
With each continued exhale, it brings to you to a place of calm and peace.

Imagine the breath brings in a glow of warmth, allowing your muscles to relax even further.
Feel the warmth traveling from the feet to the legs into the torso and hips
We become warm and heavy and relaxed
Feel warmth in the shoulders, arms, elbows, wrists, and hands
Warmth travels into our neck and face and into the crown of the head

          Warm   Calm   Relaxed   Content

Let the following imagery drift through your mind:
A meal made by a loved one
A soft comfortable sofa
blankets
Cozy socks
An open fire
A soft scarf
Roasted chestnuts
Sweet cookies
A steaming bowl of soup
Rain on the windows
Frost on the grass
Wearing slippers and pajamas
Gentle glow of fairy lights and candles
Comforting smells of cinnamon and peppermint
Holding hands
Warm hugs
Imagine yourself in your most warm and cozy place. Either real or imagined
Anywhere you can feel cozy and safe
Take a deep breath. Rub the hands together creating some warmth, and open the eyes

Hands at heart center. Namaste

Easy Pose Twist
Sun Salutation B   repeat x 3

Move Chill Yoga
Portable Yoga Class Plan 7
colder seasons

- Mountain Pose
- Chair Pose
- Standing forward fold
- Half standing forward fold
- Plank Pose
- Upward dog
- Downward dog
- Warrior I (right leg back)
- Low plank
- Upward dog
- Downward dog
- Warrior I (left leg back)
- Low plank
- Upward dog
- Downward dog
- Half standing forward fold
- Forward fold
- Chair Pose
- Mountain Pose

Revolved Reclined Dancer variation Right & Left
Hug knees in / Windshield Wiper legs

Firelog Pose RIGHT ankle over left knee	**Firelog Pose LEFT ankle over right knee**
Staff Pose	**Staff Pose**
Table Pose	
Downward Dog	**Downward Dog**
Low Lunge RIGHT foot forward	**Low Lunge Left forward**
Hamstring stretch	**Hamstring Stretch**
Mountain Pose to Standing Forward Bend	**Mountain Pose to Standing Forward Bend**

Downward Dog

Mountain Pose	**Mountain Pose**
Tree Pose RIGHT leg lifted	**Tree LEFT leg lifted**
Tree Twist / Tree Bend	**Tree Twist / Tree Bend**

Mountain Pose to Standing Forward Bend

High Lunge RIGHT leg back	**High Lunge LEFT leg back**
Crescent Twist RIGHT leg back	**Crescent Twist LEFT leg back**
Warrior I	**Warrior I**
Warrior II	**Warrior II**
Plank to Cobra	**Plank to Cobra**
Downward Dog	**Downward Dog**
Forward Fold to Mountain	**Forward Fold to Mountain**

High Lunge RIGHT foot forward	**High Lunge LEFT forward**
High Lunge Twist RIGHT	**High Lunge Twist LEFT**
Warrior I	**Warrior I**
Pyramid	**Pyramid**
Plank to Cobra	**Plank to Cobra**
Downward Dog	**Downward Dog**
Forward fold to Mountain	**Forward Fold to Mountain**

Chair to Elevated Chair
Yogi Squat
Hero Pose Stretch Right & Left
Downward Dog
Dolphin Pose to Sphinx Pose
Half Bow RIGHT and LEFT
Hero to Reclined Hero Pose
Hero to Reclined Butterfly Pose
Dead Bug
Relaxation Pose

warmer seasons

Opening Meditation
pyramid visualization

Warmer seasons bring longer days and more activity. Stay hydrated; consume larger quantities of fruits, vegetables, and yogurt. Eat vegetables and fruits that have a high water content: melons, cucumbers, and leafy greens.
This practice focuses on gentle yoga poses to balance the mind and body. Longer Savasana and meditation are especially beneficial in warmer seasons.

Sit in **Hero Pose** Virasana (VEER-AHS-uh-nuh) Kneeling on the floor, sit on the heels.
Start with **Kapalabhati Breathing** or Skull Cleanser, this technique is a cleansing breath exercise that raises your energy level dramatically.
Raise your arms straight up above your head (this promotes lymph circulation through the upper body).
Place hands in your lap and hold your hands in **Apana Mudra** for invoking the future.

Close the eyes. Inhale and fill your body with cool air. Exhale dramatically.
Repeat the same inhale and exhale several times.

Move to **Half Pyramid Pose** Ardha Parsvottanasana
(Ar-dah PARZH-voh-tahn-AHS-uh-nuh)
Keep left knee where it is in Hero Pose and extend RIGHT foot forward, pointing toes up toward head. Inhale and extend arms forward in line with the ears. Exhale bring palms to the floor framing the right shin/heel/foot, where there is a comfortable stretch. Aim to touch forehead to shinbone.
Close your eyes and take a few long, deep breaths. Begin to imagine an Egyptian pyramid. Let its image slowly take shape in your mind.
Now begin to feel yourself as this pyramid. Your legs and hips are the strong base. Your shoulders and arms the steep slopes. Your head the highest point.
Transition back to **Hero Pose** Virasana and switch legs, moving to **Half Pyramid Pose** Ardha Parsvottanasana extending LEFT foot forward. Inhale and extend arms forward in line with the ears. Exhale bring palms to the floor framing the left shin/heel/foot.
Close your eyes and take a few long, deep breaths.

As you begin to embody this pyramid, invite feelings of stability, strength, balance and quietude into your body and mind. Feel an inner settling taking place.
What would it be like to be perfectly still, solid, for thousands/millions of years?
How about sixty seconds?
Sit with this visualization for a moment; bring your attention to the breath.
Affirm to yourself – "I AM GROUNDED, I AM SECURE ,I AM MY OWN HOME."

Half Lord of the Fishes Pose Ardha Matsyendrasana
(ARD-uh MAHT-see-ehn-DRAHS-uh-nuh) In a seated position, shift your hips to the right and place your left foot just outside of your right knee, sole of the foot on the floor. Use your left fingertips to gently push into the floor behind you as you lengthen your spine. Cross your right elbow outside of your left knee, exhale and twist to the left. Come back to center. Repeat in the opposite direction.
Shift your hips to the left and place your right foot just outside of your left knee, sole of the foot on the floor. Use your left fingertips to gently push into the floor behind you as you lengthen your spine. Cross your left elbow outside of your right knee, exhale and twist to the right.

Reclined Hamstring Stretch
Supta Padangustasana Prep (soup-TAH pod-ang-goosh-TAHS-anna)
Lie back on the floor, legs extended. Exhale, bend the right knee, and draw the thigh into your torso. Hug the thigh to your belly. Press the left leg heavily to the floor, and push actively through the left heel. Hold the right leg or foot, extending the leg strait up for the stretch.

Reclining Hand to Big Toe Pose Supta Padangustasana
(SOOP-tah pahd-ahng-goosh-TAHS-uh-nuh)
Inhale and straighten the right knee, pressing the right heel up toward the ceiling. Walk your hands up the leg and reach for the inside of the big toe, elbows fully extended. Broaden the shoulder blades across your back. Press the shoulder blades lightly into the floor. Widen the collarbones. Aim to draw the foot a little closer to your head, increasing the stretch on the back of the leg.

Repeat: **Reclined Hamstring Stretch** Supta Padangustasana Prep with the LEFT leg
Repeat: **Reclining Hand to Big Toe Pose** Supta Padangustasana with the LEFT leg

Moon Salutation variation Chandra Namaskara (SHAHN-drah nah-muh-SKAR-uh)
A sequence to create a cooling flow of movement.
Unlike Sun Salutations, which are heating and stimulating, Moon Salutations Chandra Namaskara are cooling and quieting. They are used to calm the mind and draw your awareness inward. A perfect sequence when energy or temperatures are high and a tranquil, calm presence is desired.

- Mountain Pose Tadasana (Ta-DAHS-un-nah) hands at heart center
- Upward Salute Urdhva Hastasana (Oord-vah hahs-TAHS-anna)
- Standing Forward Bend Uttanasana (Oo-tan-AHS-un-nah)
- Yogi Squat Malasana (ma-LAHS-ah-nah)
- Low Lunge Right Leg Back raise arms Anjaneyasana (AHN-jah-nay-AHS-uh-nuh)
- Downward Dog Adho Mukha Svanasana (ahdo mookuh shvan-AHS-uh-na)
- Cobra Pose Bhujangasana (boo-jahn-GAHS-uh-nuh)
- Crocodile Pose Makarasana (mah-kar-AHS-uh-nuh)
- Cobra Pose Bhujangasana
- Downward Dog Adho Mukha Svanasana
- Low Lunge Left Foot Back raise arms Anjaneyasana
- Yogi Squat Malasana
- Standing Forward Bend Uttanasana
- Upward Salute Urdhva Hastasana
- Mountain Pose Tadasana hands at heart center

Repeat X3

From **Mountain Pose** Tadasana,
Move to **Standing Hand to Big Toe Pose** Utthita Hasta Padangusthasana
(oo-TEE-tah HAHS-tuh pahd-ahng-goosh-TAHS-uh-nuh)
Lifting RIGHT leg, shift the weight to your left foot
Draw your right knee up toward your chest. Loop your index and middle fingers around your right foot's big toe. Place your left hand on your left hip.
Straighten your spine. Strongly engage your abdominal muscles. Straighten your left leg, but do not lock your knee. Breathe. On an exhalation, extend and straiten your right leg forward as much as possible.
Keep both hips squared, neck and shoulders relaxed. Gaze forward.
Release by hugging the knee into your chest, and placing it down.
Stand in **Mountain Pose** Tadasana
Extend your arms sideways to shoulder-height, palms facing down.
Extended Side Angle Pose Utthita Parsvakonasana
(oo-TEE-tah PARZH-vuh-ko-NAHS-uh-nuh)
RIGHT leg back, step your feet apart in a wide stance. Bend your left knee until your left thigh is parallel to the floor, left knee directly over your heel. Keep your back leg straight. Keep your torso open to the right side space. Lower your left forearm to rest on your left thigh.
Reach your right arm up towards the ceiling, and then extend your arm over the top of your head. Right bicep covering right ear. Turn your head to look up at the ceiling.
*To deepen the pose, lower your front hand to the floor, placing your palm next to the inside arch of your front foot.
Press through both feet and come up to
Triangle Pose Utthita Trikonasana (oo-TEE-tah tree-koh-NAH-suh-nuh)
Turn your left foot out 90 degrees so your toes are pointing to the top of the mat. Pivot your right foot slightly inwards, back toe at a 45-degree angle.
Raise your arms to the sides shoulder-height and parallel to the floor. Palms facing down.
Fold at your left hip, tipping like a teapot and as if you are moving between 2 planes of glass.
Rest your left hand on your outer shin or ankle. If you are more flexible, place your right fingertips or palm on the floor to the outside of your right shin. *You can also place your hand on a block. Gaze up at right fingertips reaching toward the sky.
Release arms down, shift both feet to face the right side space and fold forward with a flat back into **Standing Straddle / Dragonfly Pose** Prasarita Padottanasana (prah-suh-REE-tuh pah-doh-tahn-AHS-uh-nuh)
Reach to rest the fingertips or palms to the mat. Lengthen through the tailbone and the crown of your head. Lengthening the spine in opposite directions. Hold and breathe.
Place the hands down to the front of mat, moving into **Plank Pose** Kumbhakasana
(koom-bahk-AHS-uh-nuh)

Shift the weight on the left hand for **Side Plank** Vasistasana
(VAH-shees-THAH-suh-nuh) with RIGHT leg pointing up in a **Tree Pose** position
Vasisthasana/Vrikshasana

Release to **Downward Dog** Adho Mukha Svanasana
(AH-doh MOO-kah-shvah-Nahs-ana)

Extend the RIGHT leg upward while bending it at the knee into

Three-legged Dog Tri Pada Adho Mukha Svanasana
(Tri-Pah-do Ah-doh MOO-kuh shvan-AHS-uh-nuh)

Walk the feet in for **Mountain Pose** Tadasana

Move to **Standing Hand to Big Toe Pose** Utthita Hasta Padangusthasana (oo-TEE-tah HAHS-tuh pahd-ahng-goosh-TAHS-uh-nuh)

Lifting LEFT leg, shift the weight to your right foot

Draw your left knee up toward your chest. Loop your index and middle fingers around your left foot's big toe. Place your right hand on your right hip.

Straighten your spine. Strongly engage your abdominal muscles. Straighten your right leg, but do not lock your knee. Breathe. On an exhalation, extend and straiten your left leg forward as much as possible.

Keep both hips squared, neck and shoulders relaxed. Gaze forward.

Release by hugging the knee into your chest, and placing it down.

Stand in **Mountain Pose** Tadasana

Extend your arms sideways to shoulder-height, palms facing down.

Extended Side Angle Pose Utthita Parsvakonasana
(oo-TEE-tah PARZH-vuh-ko-NAHS-uh-nuh)

LEFT leg back, step your feet apart in a wide stance. Bend your right knee until your right thigh is parallel to the floor, right knee directly over your heel. Keep your back leg straight. Keep your torso open to the left side space. Gaze out across the top of your right middle finger.

Lower your right forearm to rest on your right thigh.

Reach your left arm up towards the ceiling, and then extend your arm over the top of your head. Left bicep covering left ear. Turn your head to look up at the ceiling.

*To deepen the pose, lower your front hand to the floor, placing your palm next to the inside arch of your front foot.

Press through both feet and come up to

Triangle Pose Utthita Trikonasana (oo-TEE-tah tree-koh-NAH-suh-nuh)

Turn your right foot out 90 degrees so your toes are pointing to the top of the mat. Pivot your left foot slightly inwards, back toe at a 45-degree angle.

Raise your arms to the sides shoulder-height and parallel to the floor. Palms facing down.

Fold at your right hip, tipping like a teapot and as if you are moving between 2 planes of glass.

Rest your right hand on your outer shin or ankle. If you are more flexible, place your left fingertips or palm on the floor to the outside of your left shin. *You can also place your hand on a block. Gaze up at right fingertips reaching toward the sky.

Release arms down, shift both feet to face the left side space and fold forward with a flat back into **Standing Straddle / Dragonfly Pose** Prasarita Padottanasana. Reach to rest the fingertips or palms to the mat. Lengthen through the tailbone and the crown of your head. Lengthening the spine in opposite directions.
Placing hands down to front of mat, move into **Plank Pose** Kumbhakasana
Shift the weight on the left hand for **Side Plank** with LEFT leg pointing up in a **Tree Pose** position Vasisthasana/Vrikshasana
Release to **Downward Dog** Adho Mukha Svanasana (AH-doh MOO-kah-shvah-Nahs-ana) Extend the LEFT leg upward while bending it at the knee into **Three-legged Dog** Adho Mukha Svanasana
Back to **Downward Dog** Adho Mukha Svanasana

Place the Forearms to the mat and coming into **Dolphin Pose** Makarasana (makar-AHS-uh-nuh) Hold and breathe.
Lower the legs down for **Sphinx Pose** Salamba Bhujangasana (sah-LOM-bah boo-jahn-GAHS-uh-nuh) keeping the forearms flat on the mat.
Lift the head and chest, press pubic bone to the mat and strongly engage the legs.
Transition to **Seal Pose** Bhujangasana (boo-jan-GAHS-ah-nuh) by fully extending/straitening the arms, moving the hands closer toward the body any amount that allows for a comfortable amount of sensation to the lumbar spine.

Release down and bring arms behind the back, interlocking the hands.
Unsupported Cobra Pose Niralamba Bhujungasana (neera-LAM-ba boo-jahn-GAHS-uh-nuh)
Place the forehead on the ground. On an inhale, lift the chin, shoulders, chest and abdomen.
Slowly stretch and lift back with the help of the arms and the back muscles. Front body comes off the mat. Breathe. Inhale and while exhaling, slowly lower the abdomen, chest and chin to ground. Release the arms to the sides. Repeat.

Broken Wing Pose Eka Bhuja Swastikasana (eeka boo-ja swasti-KAHS-ah-na)
Lying face down, extend the right arm out to the side, palm facing down. Place the left hand under the left shoulder and gently roll onto the right hip to stretch and target the inner right arm and the chest. Legs may be bent or strait. Continue to support the upper body with your left hand. Gently lower the front body down. Repeat.
Extend the left arm out to the side, palm facing down. Place the right hand under the right shoulder and gently roll onto the left hip to stretch and target the inner left arm and the chest. Legs may be bent or strait. Continue to support the upper body with your right hand. Gently lower down.
Repeat.
Push back to sit on your heels in **Child's Pose** Balasana (bah-LAHS-ah-nuh)
Extend arms out in front on the mat, melt heart down, place forehead to mat. Option: knees apart

Come to a seated position with the soles of the feet together.
Cobbler's Pose/Bound Ankle Pose Baddha Konasana
(BAH-duh cone-AHS-uh-nuh)
*You can place blocks beneath your knees for additional support. Let knees drop to both sides. Clasp big toes with thumb and first finger. Extend the length of your entire spine skyward. Hold for 5-7 counts of breath.

Revolved Abdomen Pose Jathara Parivartanasana (jah-TAHR-uh PAHR-ee-vahr-tah-NAHS-uh-nuh)
Lie on your back with your knees bent and your feet flat on the floor.
Extend your arms out to a T, palms facing down. Straighten your legs, reaching your heels up toward the ceiling. Align your heels directly over your hips. Keep your knees soft and slightly bent.
Keep the low back flat on the floor. On an exhalation, lower both legs to the RIGHT, twisting your spine and allowing your left hip to lift all the way off the floor. Allow the force of gravity to drop your legs all the way down to the right, right foot resting on the floor. Flex your feet and stack the outer edge of your left ankle on top of your right.
Turn your head to the left and gaze toward your left hand. Keep your shoulder blades pressing down toward the floor and away from your ears.
Hold and breathe. On an inhalation, slowly come back to center, raising your feet straight up to the ceiling. Bend your knees and hug them to your chest.

Again heels up toward the ceiling, knees soft and slightly bent.
Low back flat on the floor. On an exhalation, lower both legs to the LEFT, twisting your spine and allowing your right hip to lift all the way off the floor. Allow the force of gravity to drop your legs all the way down to the left, left foot resting on the floor. Flex your feet and stack the outer edge of your right ankle on top of your left.
Turn your head to the right and gaze toward your right hand. Keep your shoulder blades pressing down toward the floor and away from your ears.
Hold and breathe. On an inhalation, slowly come back to center, raising your feet straight up to the ceiling. Bend your knees and hug them to your chest.

Legs up the wall Pose Viparita Kaeani (VIP-uh-REE-tuh kah-RAH-nee)
Bring your legs up onto the wall using your hands for balance as you shift your weight. Lower your back to the floor and lie down. Rest your shoulders and head on the floor. Scoot the lower body and pelvis to the wall. Let your arms rest open at your sides, palms facing up. Let the thigh muscles relax dropping toward the pelvis. Hold and breathe.
Release and push yourself away from the wall and slide your legs down.

Extend legs and arms and lay flat for **Relaxation Pose** Savasana (sha-VAHS-ah-nuh)
Moving onto the back. Allow feet to flop to the sides, palms facing up. Let your breathe occur naturally. Relax the face and let your eyes drop into their sockets. Invite the quiet and peace into your mind for an extra long **Relaxation Pose** Savasana.

Closing Meditation
light visualization

Sit in any comfortable seated position.

Cooling Breath variation Sheetali Pranayama (SHEE-tali prah-nah-YAH-mah)
Make an "O" shape with your lips; inhale through the lips, exhale through the nose. Feel the cool air coming in. Feel the cool air as it moves down to the abdomen. Continue for 5 more breaths like this.

Close your eyes and let your breath occur naturally.
Imagine light coming in with the breath, coming in through the top of the head and circulating throughout every part of the body.

Imagine light surrounding your body and your home.
Visualize light coming in with every inhalation
On the exhalation, visualize light going out to the world

Imagine these items in your mind's eye as you hear them.

Sunshine reflecting on the ocean
A bright yellow star
The sunrise
A sunny beach
A crackling white sparkler
An orange and yellow flame
The sunset
A cluster of stars in the sky on a clear night
A campfire
Fireworks in the sky
The sparkle in a loved one's eyes as you notice the expression of joy on their face

As you continue to breathe, feel your warm light, and send out your warm light.

Namaste.

Move Chill Yoga
Portable Yoga Class Plan 8
warmer seasons

Half Lord of the Fishes RIGHT & LEFT
Reclined Hamstring Stretch RIGHT   **Reclined Hamstring Stretch LEFT**
Reclined Hand to Big Toe RIGHT   **Reclined Hand to Big Toe LEFT**

Moon Salutation
- Mountain Pose hands at heart center
- Upward Salute
- Standing Forward Bend
- Yogi Squat
- Low Lunge Right Leg Back raise arms
- Downward Dog
- Cobra Pose
- Crocodile Pose
- Cobra Pose
- Downward Dog
- Low Lunge Left Foot Back raise arms
- Yogi Squat
- Standing Forward Bend
- Upward Salute
- Mountain Pose hands at heart center

Repeat X 3

Standing Hand to Big Toe RIGHT   **Standing Hand to Big Toe LEFT**
Mountain Pose   **Mountain Pose**
Extended Side Angle Pose RIGHT   **Extended Side Angle Pose LEFT**
Triangle Pose   **Triangle Pose**
Standing Straddle Pose   **Standing Straddle Pose**
Plank Pose   **Plank Pose**
Side Plank with Tree RIGHT   **Side Plank with Tree LEFT**
Downward Dog   **Downward Dog**
3-leg Dog RIGHT   **3-Leg Dog LEFT**
Mountain Pose   **Back to Downward Dog**

Dolphin Pose
Sphinx Pose
Seal Pose
Unsupported Cobra
Broken Wing Pose RIGHT and LEFT
Child's Pose
Cobbler's Pose
Revolved Abdomen Pose RIGHT and LEFT
Legs up the wall Pose
Relaxation Pose

9
traditional

Opening Meditation
energizing meditation

This is a traditional and simplistic practice. You can modify this practice to fit into any amount of time (30-60 minutes). Examples: Lengthen the holding of each posture, add additional rounds of Sun Salutations, slow down and deepen the meditations. Make this practice your own.

Sit in **Lotus Pose** Padmasana (Pad MAHS-ah-nuh) -Both legs folded
if too intense, **Half Lotus** Ardha Padmasana (ar-dah Pad MAHS-ah-nuh) -One leg folded.
Bend your right knee and hug it to your chest. Then, bring your right ankle to the crease of your left hip so the sole of your right foot faces the sky. The top of your foot should rest on your hip crease.
Then, bend your left knee. Cross your left ankle over the top of your right shin. The sole of your left foot should also face upwards, and the top of your foot and ankle should rest on your hip crease. Press your sit bones toward the floor and sit up straight. Rest your hands on your knees with your palms facing up.

Let the shoulders drops back and down
Palms up to bring in energy
Hands at heart
Inhale and exhale
Become aware of each breath
Let go of any pressing thoughts for the next (amount of time)

Inhale roll shoulders up towards the ears
Exhale release them down
Hold the hands and arms out strait, away from the heart with palms connected
Inhale take arms out wide opening the heart
Exhale the hands back to center
Inhale, and on the heart opening, imagine a wave of energy enveloping the body
Exhale hands together

Now, Inhale and breathe in everything that is important to you.
On the exhale, we will chant "Om"
Chanting Om is a traditional energizing vibration
Breathe in
And exhale Om
Feel the vibration of the sound

Rub your knees, stimulating the nervous system
Rotate the hips, rotate one way and then the other
Breathe in and out

"Om"
Om is a mantra. The sound OM is a vibration. Coming from Hinduism and Yoga, the mantra is considered to have high spiritual and creative power but despite this, it is a mantra that can be recited by anyone. It's both a sound and a symbol rich in meaning and depth and when pronounced correctly it is actually AUM.

"If you want to find the secrets of the universe, think in terms of energy, frequency and vibration. The very foundations of our Universe, of matter and thought, appear to lie in sound vibration." Nikola Tesla

Sit in **Easy Pose** Sukasana (soo KAHS-ah-na) Place both hands on knees.
Neck Stretching Greeva Sanchalana (Gree-va San-CHAL-ah-nuh)
Turn side to side:
Slowly turn the head to the right 3-5 seconds, keeping the chin parallel to the floor. Then slowly bring the head back to centre 3-5 seconds. Turn your head to the left side 3-5 seconds. Then slowly bring it back to the centre 3-5 seconds.
Bend neck backward and forward:
From the centre position lower the head forward and try to touch the chin to the upper chest 3-5 seconds. Gently raise the head up 3-5 seconds. Now, bend it backward as far as it will comfortably go 3-5 seconds. Then bring it back to center 3-5 seconds.
Side to Side Bend: From the center position, bend the neck to the right side so that the right ear comes towards right shoulder 3-5 seconds. Straighten the neck back to center. Bend the neck to the left side, ear to shoulder 3-5 seconds. Back to center.

Shoulder Socket Rotation Skandha Chakra (skan-dah-CHAK-ruh)
Lift the fingers of the right hand onto the right shoulder. Lift the fingers of the left hand onto the left shoulder. Lift both elbows up creating large circular motions with the elbows while the hands stay on the shoulders. Inhale on the upward stroke, exhale on the downward stroke. Now create circles going in the opposite direction. Gently touch the elbows together in the front of the body on each rotation.

Table Pose Bharmanasana (Bar-man-AHS-un-nah)
Place arms directly under shoulders, extend the neck and allow the back to be flat. Press the tail bone towards the back wall and the crown of the head towards the front wall to lengthen the spine.

Warming up spine, move into **Cat** Marjaryasana (Mahr-jahr-ee-AHS-uh-nah)
Inhale tuck tailbone, round the back, head strait, then down.
Cow Bitilasana (Bi-til-AHS-uh-nah)
Exhale arch your back, pushing shoulders back, head comes up
Repeat Cat/Cow X3
Go at your own pace, 2 or more deep breaths

Traditional Sun Salutation Surya Namaskara (SOOR-yuh nah-muh-SKAR-uh)
- Equal standing balance Samastitihi (Sa-mahs-TEE-tee-hee)
- Upward Salute Urdhva Hastasana (Oord-vah hahs-TAHS-anna)
- Standing forward Bend Uttanasana (Oo-tan-AHS-un-nah)
- Lunge Right leg back head up Anjaneyasana (AHN-jah-nay-AHS-uh-nuh)
- Downward Dog Adho Mukha Svanasana (ahdo mookuh shvan-AHS-uh-na)
- Cobra Pose Bhujangasana (boo-jang-GAHS-uh-nah)
- Downward Dog Adho Mukha Svanasana
- Lunge Left leg back head up Anjaneyasana
- Standing Forward Bend Uttanasana
- Upward Salute Urdhva Hastasana
- Equal standing balance Samastitihi

Repeat x3 or more

Sit into **Staff Pose** Dandasana (dan-DAHS-ah-nah) with your legs out in front, arms behind you with the fingertips pointing toward the body.
Head to Knee forward bend – Janu Sirshasana (JAH-new shear-SHAHS-anna)
Inhale, bend your RIGHT knee, and draw the heel between the legs. Rest your right foot sole lightly against your inner left thigh, and lay the left leg out strait.
Press your right hand against the inner right groin, where the thigh joins the pelvis, and your left hand on the floor beside the hip. Exhale and lift the torso as you fold down with a flat back. Line up your navel with the middle of the left thigh.
*You can use a strap to help you lengthen the spine evenly and ground through the sit bones.
Then reach your left hand to the outside of the foot. With the arms fully extended.
Back to **Staff Pose** Dandasana
Head to Knee forward bend – Janu Sirshasana (JAH-new shear-SHAHS-anna)
Inhale, bend your LEFT knee, and draw the heel between the legs. Rest your left foot sole lightly against your inner right thigh, and lay the right leg out strait.
Press your left hand against the inner left groin, where the thigh joins the pelvis, and your right hand on the floor beside the hip. Exhale and lift the torso as you fold down with a flat back. Line up your navel with the middle of the right thigh.
Then reach your right hand to the outside of the foot. With the arms fully extended.

Come up to stand in **Mountain Pose** Tadasana
Lift the RIGHT leg for **Tree pose** Vrksasana (vrik-SHAH-suh-nuh)
Shifting the weight onto your left foot. Lengthen through your tailbone and through the crown of the head. Arms up, begin to tip to the right side, left arm over the left ear, bringing right arm down to rest on the right knee. Feel the stretch in your left side.

Standing Yoga Seal Dandayamana Mudrasana
(Dan-day-AHM-un-ah Mu-DRAHS-ah-nuh)
From Mountain pose, step the legs 3-4 feet apart into Five Pointed Star. Inhale the arms up and then drop them behind you. Interlace the fingers together. Draw the shoulder blades towards each other and lift the chest and gaze up towards the ceiling.
Exhale and hinge at the hips coming forward with the chest, reaching the arms up and forward. Let the head hang relaxed from the neck.

Keep the arms and legs straight. If you feel the weight back in the heels try and shift your weight forward slightly. Breathe and hold for 4-8 breaths.
Release: keep the shoulder blades squeezed together as you inhale back up, taking a deep breath into the belly and chest. Exhale release the arms.
Repeat.

Stand in **Mountain Pose** Tadasana
Lift the LEFT leg for **Tree pose** Vrksasana (vrik-SHAH-suh-nuh)
Shifting the weight onto your right foot. Lengthen through your tailbone and through the crown of the head. Arms up, begin to tip to the left side, right arm over the right ear, bringing left arm down to rest on the left knee. Feel the stretch in your right side.
Repeat the **Standing Yoga Seal** Dandayamana Mudrasana

Come down to lay on the front body. Chin to the floor, legs together and arms alongside the body. Palms facing down.
Half Locust Pose Ardha Shalabasana (Ar-duh Sha-la-BAHS-ah-nuh)
Rock the hips from side to side to walk the arms underneath your body, so the forearms are on the inside of the hip bones and the hands are under the thighs.
Inhale and lengthen the legs, reaching the toes away from your body. Pull up the knee caps, squeeze the buttocks and engage the abdominals. Press the arms down into the mat and slowly lift the legs up towards the ceiling.
Breathe and hold for 2-5 breaths. On an exhale, slowly lower the legs to the floor.

Come to kneel in **Hero Pose** Virasana (Veer AHS-ah-na)
Camel Pose Ustrasana (oosh-TRAHS-anna)
Plant your shin bones into the mat, Lift pelvis up and bend backwards while exhaling slowly. Maintaining length in the body, push pelvis forward as you place hands on lower back. Head moves back.
To go deeper, extend arms one by one pressing palms against heels.

Move to lay on the back for **Sleeping Abdominal Stretch Pose**
Supta Udarakarshanasana (soop-ta Oo-DARA-karsh-an-AHS-an-ah)
Bend the knees and bring the feet towards you with the sole of the feet resting on the floor. Keep the two feet together. Bring arms out to a T flat on the floor with palms facing up.
Exhale and turn the knees towards the RIGHT side and try to touch the right thigh to the floor. Take it as far as possible without straining. Look to your left hand. Breathe.
On an inhale, bring back the knees to the upright center position.
Repeat on left side: **Sleeping Abdominal Stretch Pose** Supta Udarakarshanasana
Bend the knees and bring the feet towards you with the sole of the feet resting on the floor. Keep the two feet together. Bring arms out to a T flat on the floor with palms facing up.
Exhale and turn the knees towards the LEFT side and try to touch the left thigh to the floor. Take it as far as possible without straining. Look to your right hand.
Breathe. On an inhale, bring back the knees to the upright center position.

Extend legs and arms and lay flat for **Relaxation Pose** Savasana (sha-VAHS-ah-nuh)
Relax the body completely for a guided Savasana.

Closing Meditation
traditional yoga nidra variation

Phase 1. Ready for Meditation
Bring your attention to the world around you. Listen to the sounds outside the room. Listen to the sounds inside the room. Allow yourself a moment to become aware of all sensations around you: sounds, smells, temperature. Visualize your own body resting on the floor, and become aware of your own physical presence.

Phase 2. Sanctuary within
Move inward for a moment and see if you can discover a retreat or sanctuary within. A place where you feel calm and secure. Perhaps there is a particular place you like to go or a person you like to be with. Spend a moment imagining this place and know that you may return to it at any time during this meditation, and surely at some time during your life, you may return to it when you need it.

Phase 3. Mindful of Body
Bring your awareness to your body in the here and now. Feel your stillness. Notice if finding stillness is easy. Notice if any specific parts of your body are more tense than others. Sense the entirety of your body all at the same time. Feel the entire physical presence of all that is you.

Phase 4. The Breath
Bring your awareness to your breath. Feel the breath entering into the body. Notice the flow into the chest and abdomen. Feel the energy of the inhale and the relaxation of the exhale. Count 10 energizing and relaxing breaths.

Phase 5. Emotions
Without evaluating or judging, acknowledge any feelings that are currently coming up for you. If you notice tension, allow yourself to feel it. Now feel the emotion that is the direct opposite to tension, or the exact opposite of anything negative that comes up for you.

Phase 6. Thoughts
Breathe. Now thoughts, memories, or images that come up for you right now. Acknowledge them. If anything negative comes to mind, think about the exact opposite of whatever that is.

Phase 7. Find Happiness
Bring to mind a memory that holds great happiness and peace for you. Then, linger here, imagining and remembering as many details as possible of this memory.

Phase 8. This practice
Reflect on how this practice has made you feel. Begin to feel your body again, becoming aware of body and breath. Become aware of the room. Let your eyes open and slowly come to a seated position.

Namaste.

Move Chill Yoga
Portable Yoga Class Plan 9
traditional

Lotus Pose/Half Lotus Pose
Easy Pose
Neck Stretching
Shoulder Socket Rotation
Table Pose
Cat Pose
Cow Pose

Sun Salutation
- Equal standing balance
- Upward Salute
- Standing forward Bend
- Right leg back head up
- Downward Dog
- Cobra
- Downward Dog
- Left leg back head up
- Standing Forward Bend
- Upward Salute
- Equal standing balance

Repeat x3 or more

Staff Pose	**Staff Pose**
Head to Knee Forward Bend RIGHT	**Head to Knee Forward Bend LEFT**
Mountain Pose	**Mountain Pose**
Tree Pose RIGHT leg	**Tree Pose LEFT leg**
Tree Pose Side Stretch RIGHT	**Tree Pose Side Stretch LEFT**
Standing Yoga Seal	**Standing Yoga Seal**

Half Locust Pose
Hero Pose
Camel Pose
Sleeping Abdominal Stretch Pose RIGHT and LEFT
Relaxation Pose

10
gratitude

Opening Meditation
being grateful

Sit in **Easy Pose** Sukhasana (Soo- KAHS-uh-nah)
Close your eyes. Connect with your breath.
Imagine breathing in a soft warm glow of yellow and orange warm light.
It feels much like the way the warm sun feels on your skin on a beautiful day.
Allow yourself to be here relaxed warm with this soft glow filling in all around you.

Let the answers to these questions float through your mind, and hold the thought until the next question.

- What made me smile today?
- What is the best thing that happened today?
- What did I see today that I liked?
- What did I hear today that I liked?
- What felt good today?
- Who or What inspired me today?

Next, bring to mind those people in your life to whom you are close: your friends, family, spouse…. Say to yourself, "For them, I am grateful."
Next, turn your attention onto yourself: you are a unique individual, blessed with imagination, the ability to communicate, to learn, to overcome. Say to yourself:
"For this, I am grateful."
Finally, rest into the realization that life is a precious gift. That you have been born into a time period of success and prosperity, we have homes, cars, clothes, the gift of life & health, doctors, culture and access to various teachings of all kinds to learn and to express ourselves, Say to yourself: "For these gifts, I am grateful."

Let you mind explore whatever else you are grateful for and truly appreciate.
Notice how you feel in this moment as you focus on the abundance of all these things.

Now imagine the energy of all your gratitude in that soft yellow orange light surrounding you.

Sun Salutation A Surya Namaskara
With Sun Salutation A, practice breathing through the nose, which warms the air, just as the **vinyasa** warms up the body. Vin-YAHS-ah - **movement/flowing sequence in coordination with the breath.**
Exhale when bending or folding and inhale when extending.

- Mountain pose Tadasana (Ta-DAHS-un-nah)
- Upward salute Urdhva Hastasana (oord-vah hahs-TAHS-anna)
- Standing forward fold Uttanasana (OO-tan-AHS-un-nah)
- Half forward fold Ardha Uttanasana (Ar-duh OO-tan-AHS-un-nah)
- High plank pose Utthita Chaturanga Dandasana into four-limbed staff pose Chaturanga Dandasana (oo-tee-tah chah-tuur-ANGH-uh dahn-DAHS-uh-nuh)
- Upward-facing dog Urdhva Mukha Svanasana (oord-vuh-Mookuh shvan-AHS-uh-na)
- Downward-facing dog Adho Mukha Svanasana (ahdo mookuh shvan-AHS-uh-na)
- Half forward fold Ardha Uttanasana
- Standing forward fold Uttanasana
- Upward salute Urdhva hastasana
- Mountain pose Tadasana

Repeat X 3

Prana (prah-nah) a life-giving force
Building prana in the chest builds buoyancy and lightness and uplifts us.
From **Mountain Pose** Tadasana hold your elbows and fold into **Standing Forward Bend** Uttanasana with a flat back.
Inhale come up with a flat back, elevating both arms overhead. Lift heels off the mat and stretch up tall. Exhale come down slowly, diving forward with a flat back. Feel the releasing in your lower back.
Inhale elevate arms overhead, lift heels off the mat, stretching up tall. Exhale fold forward.
Repeat x 6
On the last fold, stay here for 7 full breaths. Bending at the knee slightly if that feels comfortable.

Table Pose Bharmanasana (Bar-man-AHS-un-nah)
Place arms directly under shoulders, extend the neck and allow the back to be flat.
Press the tailbone towards the back wall and the crown of the head towards the front wall to lengthen the spine.
Warming up spine, move into **Cat Pose** Marjaryasana (Mahr-jahr-ee-AHS-uh-nah)
Inhale tuck tailbone, round the back.
Then, move to **Cow Pose** Bitilasana
(Bi-til-AHS-uh-nah) Exhale arch your back, pushing shoulders back, head comes up
Repeat Cat/Cow X3
Go at your own pace, 2 or more deep breaths

Tuck toes and push back to
Downward Dog Adho Mukha Svanasana (AH-doh MOO-kah-shvah-Nahs-ana)
Deep breath - All 10 fingers and palms pressing into mat, hips up as if a string is pulling up the hips, gaze at belly button. Find stillness

Step the RIGHT leg between the hands.
Extended Side Angle Pose Utthita Parsvakonasana
(oo-TEE-tah PARZH-vuh-ko-NAHS-uh-nuh)
RIGHT leg and foot/toes point to the top of your mat. Bend your right knee until your right thigh is parallel to the floor. Keep your right knee directly over your heel. Align the heel of your right foot with the arch of your left foot. Keep your back leg straight. Place your right forearm on your right knee, or right fingertips to the floor inside the arch of your right foot. Reach your left arm up towards the ceiling, and then extend your left arm over the top of your head. Left bicep over left ear, and your fingertips should be reaching in the same direction your front toes are pointing.
Turn your head to look up at the ceiling.
Building prana, Coordinate the arm movement with the breath. Inhale arm overhead, exhale take the hand back to the hip.
Repeat the arm movement x 6

Come to **Warrior I** Virabhadrasana I (Veer-ah-bah-DRAHS-ana)
Arms strait up towards the sky. Create 1 long line of energy from your back heel through the tips of your fingers.
Interlace fingers behind you. **Devotional/Humble Warrior** Baddha Virabhadrasana
(ba-DAH Veer-ah-bah-DRAHS-ana)
Inhale expanding chest and lungs. As you exhale, continue to keep your heart open and gently bow forward, while your arms extend backward and upward. The right shoulder may graze the right leg even further to the right as you release your pelvis and drop deeper into the pose.

Come up to **Mountain Pose** Tadasana
Move into **1-legged Chair Pose** Eka Pada Utkatasana (Eeka-pah-duh Oot-Kah –TAS –uh-nah)
Hugging in the right leg, resting right heel on left thigh. Bend your left knee as if sitting. Pause. Now straiten left leg.
Extend your right leg out in front, grabbing the outer edge side of the right foot with your left hand for **Revolved Hand to Big Toe** Parivrtta Hasta Padangusthasana
(Pari Vri-TUH HAHS-tuh pahd-ahng-goosh-TAHS-uh-nuh)
Twist from the waist to the right side of the space, and extend your right arm out behind. Balance. Breathe. Hug your right leg back in.
Bend your left leg, and step the right leg back to **Warrior I** Virabhadrasana I
Cartwheel arms down to frame the front foot

Tuck toes and push back to
Downward Dog Adho Mukha Svanasana
Deep breath - All 10 fingers and palms pressing into mat, hips up as if a string is pulling up the hips, gaze at belly button. Find stillness

Step the LEFT leg between the hands.
Extended Side Angle Pose Utthita Parsvakonasana
(oo-TEE-tah PARZH-vuh-ko-NAHS-uh-nuh)
LEFT leg and foot/toes point to the top of your mat. Bend your left knee until your left thigh is parallel to the floor. Keep your left knee directly over your heel. Align the heel of your left foot with the arch of your right foot. Keep your back leg straight.

Place your left forearm on your left knee, or left fingertips to the floor inside the arch of your left foot. Reach your right arm up towards the ceiling, and then extend your right arm over the top of your head. Right bicep over right ear, and your fingertips should be reaching in the same direction your front toes are pointing.
Turn your head to look up at the ceiling.
Building prana, Coordinate the arm movement with the breath. Inhale arm overhead, exhale take the hand back to the hip.
Repeat the arm movement x 6

Come up to **Warrior I** Virabhadrasana I (Veer-ah-bah-DRAHS-ana)
Arms strait up towards the sky. Create 1 long line of energy from your back heel through the tips of your fingers.
Interlace fingers behind you. **Devotional/Humble Warrior** Baddha Virabhadrasana (ba-DAH Veer-ah-bah-DRAHS-ana)
Inhale expanding chest and lungs. As you exhale, continue to keep your heart open and gently bow forward, while your arms extend backward and upward. The left shoulder may graze the left leg even further to the left as you release your pelvis and drop deeper into the pose.

Come up to **Mountain Pose** Tadasana
Move into **1-legged Chair Pose** Eka Pada Utkatasana (Eeka-pah-duh Oot-Kah –TAS –uh-nah)
Hugging in the left leg, resting left heel on right thigh. Bend your right knee as if sitting. Pause. Now straiten right leg.
Extend your left leg out in front, grabbing the outer edge side of the left foot with your right hand for **Revolved Hand to big toe** Parivrtta Hasta Padangusthasana (Pari Vri-TUH HAHS-tuh pahd-ahng-goosh-TAHS-uh-nuh)
Twist from the waist to the left side of the space, and extend your left arm out behind. Balance. Breathe. Hug your left leg back in.
Bend your right leg, and step the left leg back to **Warrior I** Virabhadrasana I
Jump or walk back to **Plank Pose** Kumbhakasana (koom-bahk-AHS-uh-nuh)
Upward Dog Urdhva Mukha Svanasana
Downward Dog Adho Mukha Svanasana
Find some stillness here for a moment.
When you are ready, come up to the front of your mat into **Mountain Pose** Tadasana for
Sun Salutation A Surya Namaskara
- Mountain pose Tadasana
- Upward salute Urdhva Hastasana
- Standing forward fold Uttanasana
- Half forward fold Ardha Uttanasana
- High plank pose Utthita Chaturanga Dandasana into four-limbed staff pose Chaturanga Dandasana
- Upward-facing dog Urdhva Mukha Svanasana
- Downward-facing dog Adho Mukha Svanasana
- Half forward fold Ardha Uttanasana
- Standing forward fold Uttanasana
- Upward salute Urdhva hastasana
- Mountain pose Tadasana

Drop knees down and push back to **Child's Pose** Balasana (bah-LAHS-ah-nuh), arms extended, forehead on mat. Stay here breathing, and allow your body to sink.

Moving the hips forward, allow the pelvis to drop to the floor into
Sphinx Pose Salamba Bhujangasana (sah-LOM-bah boo-jahn-GAHS-uh-nuh) keeping the forearms flat on the mat. Lift the head and chest, opening the heart, and press pubic bone to the mat and strongly engage the legs.
Unwind the neck here. Slowly roll your neck one way and then the other way. This brings fluid to your neck and vertebra.

As you unwind, gently lower your upper body to the ground into
Crocodile Pose Makarasana (mah-kar-AHS-uh-nuh)
Stretch out on the mat face down. Extended legs a little wider then hip distance apart. Toes turned out, heels turned in. Fold your arms and place your hands on opposite elbows. Shoulders and head are off the mat. Rest the forehead on the forearms.
Close the eyes and relax the body.

Bring the front body down flat on the mat, arms and hands to your sides for
Bow Pose Dhanurasana (DAHN-yoor-AHS-uh-nuh)
Bend your knees. Bring your heels as close as you can to your buttocks, keeping your knees hip-distance apart.
Reach back with both hands and hold onto your outer ankles.
On an inhalation, lift your heels up toward the ceiling, drawing your thighs up and off the mat. Your head, chest, and upper torso will also lift off the mat.
Gaze Forward and extend and lift a little higher.
Release down. Still holding your ankles, tip the body down to the right so your heart is open to the left side of the space and your right shoulder, and right side body are on the mat. Hold for 5 breath counts.
Come back to center. Still holding your ankles, tip the body down to the left so your heart is open to the right side of the space and your left shoulder, and left side body are on the mat. Hold for 5 breath counts.

Release down to **Locust Pose** Shalabasana (shah-lah-BAHS-uh-nuh)
Rest your forehead on the mat, extending legs strait behind. Press your weight evenly across tops of both feet. With arms alongside the body, inhale look forward lifting your chest and arms. Widen across the collar bones. Then, lift the feet off the mat. Hold and breathe. Release down. Repeat.

Push back to sit on your heels in **Child's Pose** Balasana (bah-LAHS-ah-nuh)
Extend arms out in front on the mat, melt heart down, place forehead to mat. Option: knees apart. Continue to sink down even further.

Transition to the back, laying on the mat with your knees bent and touching. Feet parallel and aligned with hips. Draw your heels closer to your tailbone.

Upward Bow / Wheel Pose Urdhva Dhanurasana (OORD-vuh DAHN-yoor-AHS-uh-nuh)
Reach your arms up overhead, and then bend your elbows so that you can place your palms on the floor at either side of your head. Keep your forearms parallel as you extend your fingers toward your heels. Reach your elbows directly up toward the ceiling.
Inhale as you press your feet firmly into the floor and lift your hips upward toward the ceiling. Contract your abdominal muscles and thighs to support your lower back. Press through the palms of your hands and lift your shoulders off the mat.
Hold for a few breaths.
On an exhalation, straighten your arms and lift your head completely off the floor. Press the weight of your hands equally through your index fingers. Draw your chest toward the wall closest to your head. *Do not rest your weight on your head or the neck. As you practice and gain strength and flexibility, you will be able to lift your head off the mat easier each time.
Lift your chest even more toward the wall behind you. Straighten your arms and legs even more. Broaden your shoulder blades across your back. Let your head hang. Gaze at the floor between your hands.
Hold for up to 20 breaths. Release the pose by gently touching the crown of your head to the mat, and then your whole body. Rest on your back with your knees bent.

With an exhale, bend your knees into the belly for
Happy Baby Pose Ananda Balasana (ah-NAND-ah Bah-LAHS-ah-nuh)
Hold the outsides of the feet, open knees slightly wider than your torso and bring them toward your armpits. Ankles align over the knees, flex the heels. Push your feet into the hands to create a little resistance. Lower the sacrum into the mat.

Release legs down again so the knees are touching and bent. Rest your arms at your sides. Cross the right ankle over the left knee to rest on the left thigh.
Reverse Pigeon Pose variation Sucirandhrasana (Soo-kee-ran-DRHAS-ah-nuh)
Thread your hands through your thighs holding the back of the left (lower) thigh. Gently pull the left thigh towards you, raising the foot off the floor. Keep the foot flexed. Hold and breathe.
Release the legs down, rest your arms at your sides. Cross the left ankle over the right knee to rest on the right thigh.
Thread your hands through your thighs holding the back of the right (lower) thigh. Gently pull the right thigh towards you, raising the foot off the floor. Keep the foot flexed. Hold and breathe.

Release the entire body down for **Relaxation Pose** Savasana (sha-VAHS-ah-nuh)
Allow legs to fall naturally to the sides. Eyes closed and relaxed.

Closing Meditation
sharing gratitude

Take a comfortable seated position, or remain laying in **Relaxation Pose** Savasana
Focus inward and downward toward your heart.

Close your eyes.
Notice the breath moving in and out without any effort required
Feel grateful for each breath.
Notice the way your heart is beating without any effort.
Feel grateful for each heartbeat and each heartbeat you've been blessed with
so far in your life.
Notice your mind.
Feel grateful for the amazing human mind that can observe, dream, believe, and learn.
Feel grateful for your minds.
Notice your senses.
Hearing, Sight, Smell, Taste, Touch - all of which help us to enjoy our lives.
Feel grateful for each one.
Think about where we sleep at night.
Feel grateful for having somewhere to call home.
Friends, Family members, and people we feel blessed to have in our lives.
Feel what gratitude feels like and imagine it is that soft orange yellow light.
Feel it's warmth, feel it growing a little more as you keep all these things we are
grateful for in our minds.
Imagine all these gifts and people you are grateful for in a circle around you.
Now imagine the orange yellow light and warmth surrounding those people also.
Allow the light of gratitude to expand to embrace people in your life that you might find
not so pleasant or tricky or challenging.
Imagine this light and wellbeing filling and surrounding these people. Transform their
expressions into happiness.
Now Imagine this light to encompass all beings – people you haven't met yet - and animals..
plants.. all warmed by your light and energy of your gratitude.

Imagine being held in a circle a lot like the inside of an egg
You are inside your egg of gratitude energy, light and warmth.
Notice again your breath. The ground firm beneath you.
When you are ready gently open your eyes.
If you are laying down, come up and roll onto one side.

Namaste

Move Chill Yoga
Portable Yoga Class Plan 10
gratitude

Sun Salutation A
- Mountain Pose
- Upward Salute
- Standing Forward Fold
- Half Forward Fold
- High Plank Pose
- Upward Dog Pose
- Downward Dog Pose
- Half Forward Fold
- Standing Forward Fold
- Upward Salute
- Mountain Pose

Repeat X 3

Building Prana: Mountain Pose/Standing Forward Bend x 6

Table
Cat Pose and Cow Pose x 3
Downward Dog

Extended Side Angle Pose RIGHT	Extended Side Angle LEFT
Warrior I	Warrior I
Devotional Warrior	Devotional Warrior
Mountain Pose	Mountain Pose
1-Leg Chair Pose RIGHT	1-Leg Chair Pose LEFT
Revolved Hand to big toe RIGHT	Revolved Hand to big toe LEFT
Warrior I	Warrior I
Downward Dog	Plank Pose

Sun Salutation A
- Mountain Pose
- Upward Salute
- Standing Forward Fold
- Half Forward Fold
- High Plank Pose
- Upward Dog Pose
- Downward Dog Pose
- Half Forward Fold
- Standing Forward Fold
- Upward Salute
- Mountain Pose

Repeat X 3

Child's Pose
Sphinx Pose / Unwind the neck
Crocodile Pose

Bow Pose
Bow Pose RIGHT & LEFT
Locust Pose
Child's Pose
Upward Bow/Wheel
Happy Baby Pose
Reverse Pigeon Pose variation RIGHT & LEFT
Relaxation Pose

11

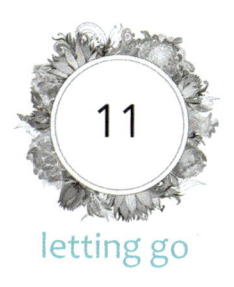

letting go

Opening Meditation
spine visualization

Begin in **Easy Pose** Sukhasana (Soo- KAHS-uh-nah),
Close your eyes. Rest hands lightly on the knees. Gently press through the tailbone.
Imagine your spine inside the body. Imagine the tailbone resting on the mat, and imagine the length of the spine all the way up to the crown of the head.
Now imagine the spine is an elevator with a car that can travel up and down.
Imagine this elevator car at your tailbone or the "basement".
Think of a few things that maybe troubled you this week, maybe these things are sitting in the basement. Maybe you are still holding onto them.
Imagine those thoughts or things getting inside the elevator car at the basement, at your tailbone. Feel the elevator rise from the basement, taking all these unwanted thoughts and things up with it.

INHALE Let the elevator reach the top of your head or "the roof terrace".
Imagine all these unwanted thoughts and things getting off at the roof terrace as you EXHALE. Now let the elevator car travel back down your spine.
INHALE let the elevator car pick up anything negative and unwanted it might have left behind. Let it float again all the way up to the roof terrace and EXHALE all the negative things out. See them get off the elevator and disappear out into the clouds as you breathe out.
This time, the elevator car stays up on the roof terrace. Pause and breathe a few times.
Now imagine a number of beautiful things getting on the elevator.
Laughter, Smiles, Happiness, Confidence, Comfort, Warmth, Energy…
Now let the elevator car move freely and easily up and down spreading all the positive thoughts throughout your body.

Easy Alternate Nostril Breathing Nadi Shodhana (NAH-dee shoh-DAH-nuh)
This is a purifying pranayama where we alternate the blockage of each nostril. This concentrates the flow of the breath throughout the body.
It balances energy throughout the body, and makes connections with the left and right sides of the brain. This is an effective form of pranayama that will ease stress and relax the body.
To begin, make the hang loose sign with the right hand. Place your thumb on your right nostril, closing the right nostril. Take three easy inhale and exhales with the right nostril closed, breathing through the left nostril only.

Place your pinky on your left nostril, closing the left nostril. Take three easy inhale and exhales with the left the nostril closed, using the right nostril only.
Feel the breath going all the way down. Repeat right and left.

We all need to slow down and let go.
This is a long hold Hatha sequence that invites you to further let go into each posture. It will unravel additional layers of strength that you didn't know existed. You may notice movement of your mind inside stillness of the body.
Pay attention to your breath see what comes up for you.
Hold each posture for 10 breath counts. 10 inhale/exhales.

Begin in **Child's Pose** Balasana (bah-LAHS-ah-nuh)
Find comfort and surrender. Let your knees be wide or together.
Extend arms out, melt heart down, place forehead to mat.
Inhale a sense of light and expansiveness. Exhale chaos and disorder.
Soften face go a little deeper. Create space in the body so it can fill with limitless possibilities.

Downward Dog Adho Mukha Svanasana
(AH-doh MOO-kah-shvah-Nahs-ana)
Find the pose and try not to adjust. Try to enjoy the space of the posture and how it feels. Maybe the alignment is not perfect. That is ok. Just surrender to what you've given yourself, right here and now. Inhale light and space. Exhale disorder and dark.

Step into **Standing Forward Bend** Uttanasana (OO-tan-AHS-un-nah)
Find where your hands will be comfortable. At your knees, at your shins or ankles. If you are more flexible, the floor. *Place blocks under your hands, or bend the knees slightly I that works for you. Choose how it feels good and then stay with it.
Let go of that which distracts us.

Bend the legs inhale into **Chair Pose** Utkatasana (OOT-kuh-TAHS-uh-nuh)
Choose "cactus" arms or hands together at heart center. Be here with intention in the posture. Feel your body being challenged and breathe into the spots that need strength.

Inhale stand float arms to your sides **Mountain Pose** Tadasana (Ta-DAHS-un-nah)
Try to feel a sense of ease as you hold Mountain Pose. Feel the steadiness of your own space. Feel satisfaction being right here right now.

Step any leg back into **Warrior II** Virabhadrasana II (Veer-ah-bah-DRAHS-ana)
Feel space and let go of tension. Feel ease in this posture. Feel your bones within you supporting your body. Inhale happiness, exhale tension.

Slowly straiten your leg and back to **Mountain Pose** Tadasana

Warrior II Virabhadrasana II to the other side.
Close eyes and feel. Just enjoy the experience of you.

Triangle Pose Utthita Trikonasana (oo-TEE-tah tree-koh-NAH-suh-nuh)
Find yourself in this pose. If it's too much to hold the gaze up, then look forward.
Inhale possibility, exhale distractions. Rest in this moment.

Back to **Mountain Pose** Tadasana
Feel the space inside you. Trust yourself on your own 2 feet.

Triangle Pose Utthita Trikonasana to the other side.
Soften the mind. Breathe in clarity, exhale messiness.

Mountain Pose Tadasana
Take another long moment here to feel steadiness. Soften your heart.

Wide Leg Forward Fold
Prasarita Padottanasana (prah-suh-REE-tuh pah-doh-tahn-AHS-uh-nuh)
Inhale lengthen the torso as you fold at the hips. Bring hands where comfortable.
Or, place blocks under your head or under your hands.
Release from your lower back.
Try to get the inside stillness to match your outside stillness in this pose.

High Plank Kumbhakasana (koom-bahk-AHS-uh-nuh)
Feel how can you find stillness in your plank.
Make the body light. Inhale making more space in the body, exhale releasing negativity.
Allow yourself to not adjust physically. Face your own mind and hold.

Slowly lower to **Crocodile Pose** Makarasana (mah-kar-AHS-uh-nuh)
Relax all tension. Find stillness.

Locust Pose Shalabasana (shah-lah-BAHS-uh-nuh)
Holding this pose for 2-5 minutes is wonderful for your mind. Breathe and hold.

Child's Pose Balasana
Let yourself feel what this practice did for you.
A lot of yogis find that long hold practices are their favorite practices.

Bow Pose Dhanurasana (DAHN-yoor-AHS-uh-nuh)
Release to lay on your front body. If your hip bones bother you, you can place a blanket under the hip points. Reach around with both hands to hold the ankles. Open the heart and reach upward with the legs. Feel the light and steady quality inside. Begin to glow from the inside out.

Crocodile Pose Makarasana
Feel the luxury of your own space. Breathe in beauty, exhale anything you no longer need. Begin to notice in your mind if something has changed.

Release legs down into **Relaxation Pose** Savasana (sha-VAHS-ah-nuh)
Commit to total physical stillness. Feel the weight of your bones on the floor. Give into gravity. Give into the fact that the universe and something bigger than us has a part in our life. Feel any sense of doubt or fear or insecurity disappear. (stay in Shavasana for at least 15-20 counts of breath)
Slowly roll your hips side to side, your head side to side. Move to one side and come up.

Closing Meditation
the disappearing jar

Sit in Easy Pose Sukhasana (Soo- KAHS-uh-nah)
Close your eyes and sit up tall. This is an excellent and effective visualization you can use to help remove any overwhelming stresses that are causing issue for you in mind and body.

Imagine a large plain glass jar. Open the jar with your mind and picture yourself putting all your stresses and problems inside. Close the jar and seal it very tightly. So tightly that it cannot be opened again.

Now imagine the jar shrinking down in size. As it gets smaller and smaller you are helping to effectively put these stresses and problems in perspective.

Continue to mentally shrink down the jar until the jar has disappeared.
This is an exercise you can visualize everyday. We can learn that problems and stresses are sometimes only as big as we picture them.

Long Hold Practice – hold each posture for at least 10 breath counts

Child's Pose
Downward Dog
Standing Forward Bend
Chair Pose
Mountain Pose
Warrior II
Mountain Pose
Warrior II
Triangle Pose
Mountain Pose
Triangle Pose
Mountain Pose
Wide Leg Forward Fold
High Plank
Crocodile Pose
Locust Pose
Child's Pose
Bow Pose
Crocodile Pose
Relaxation Pose

Move Chill Yoga
Portable Yoga Class Plan 11
letting go

12
strength & balance

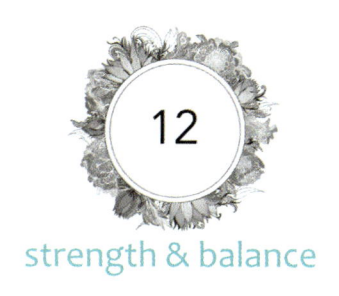

Opening Meditation
sphere in the sand

Begin in **Easy Pose** Sukhasana (Soo- KAHS-uh-nah),

Transport yourself to a tropical sandy coastline.
Imagine bending down and with your hand or fingers, draw a sphere in the sand that completely surrounds where you are seated. The sphere in the sand represents a safe boundary. No one can cross into it, and you are not expected to step out of the sphere.
You are creating a boundary.

Now broaden your boundary. Imagine standing up and stepping out of the sphere. The ocean tides are coming to shore and washing away your drawn sphere.
Now move back and draw a new much larger sphere that gives you even more space for growth and expression. More space to be you.

Now imagine the line of the large sphere fading slowly into the sand.
You can still see the boundary, but it allows you to breathe, expand, and grow even more. It allows representations of what you love to come into your space as you wish.

Take a few deep breaths while you visualize being on this tropical sandy beach.

This sequence is about tapping into the core of who you are so you can navigate this life with a stronger sense of self. The movements in this sequence will help to strengthen your center so you can begin to live from it—lift yourself up, and ultimately those around you. It can be used as an ongoing practice, incorporated into your regular routine, or can be called upon when you feel you need to speak up or ask your inner voice for guidance.

Start sitting on heels in **Diamond Pose** Vajrasana (vahj-RAHS-uh-nuh)
Round and arch the spine 3 to 5 times, activating your connection with the breath.

Press hands to the mat into **Table Pose** Bharmanasana (Bar-man-AHS-un-nah)
Dancing Cat /Moving Balancing Table variation
(dan-day-AHM-na bar-man-AHS-ah-nah)
Inhale and extend the RIGHT arm and left leg. Breathe and hold. Then, round the back and exhale drawing the knee to nose and placing the right hand back down on the mat. Repeat the sequence 5 times, using the inhale to extend the leg, and the exhale to draw the knee in towards the nose. Press firmly into the right shin and left hand on the mat.
Inhale and extend the LEFT arm and right leg. Breathe and hold. Then, round the back and exhale drawing the knee to nose and placing the left hand back down on the mat. Repeat the sequence 5 times, using the inhale to extend the leg, and the exhale to draw the knee in towards the nose. Press firmly into the left shin and right hand on the mat.

Revolving Planks
Lie on your RIGHT side on the mat with the right forearm and elbow flat on the mat. Stack together your legs, knees, ankles and feet. Tighten abs.
Push your right elbow and hand against the floor as you lift up your glutes and hips off the floor until right shoulder, right hip, and right foot are in a straight line. Reach up with your left hand and extend.
Rotate your torso downwards and reach under your body with your left arm to a traditional **Plank Pose** Kumbhakasana (koom-bahk-AHS-uh-nuh). Rotate back to the side plank with left arm up and repeat for 10-12 times before switching sides.
*Take a modification with the knee on the mat as you work to find strength and stability.
Switch Sides: Lie on your LEFT side on the mat with the left forearm and elbow flat on the mat. Stack together your legs, knees, ankles and feet. Tighten abs.
Push your left elbow and hand against the floor as you lift up your glutes and hips off the floor until left shoulder, left hip, and left foot are in a straight line. Reach up with your right hand and extend.
Rotate your torso downwards and reach under your body with your right arm to a traditional **Plank Pose** Kumbhakasana. Rotate back to the side plank with right arm up and repeat for 10-12 times
*Take a modification with the knee on the mat as you work to find strength and stability.

Tuck toes and push up to **Downward Dog** Adho Mukha Svanasana (AH-doh MOO-kah-shvah-Nahs-ana) Raise pelvis skyward, pressing through all 10 fingers and palms. Head is relaxed. Gaze at the core.

Dancing Dog
Down Dog Split RIGHT LEG Tri Pada Adho Mukha Svanasana (Tri Pada AH-doh MOO-kah-shvah-Nahs-ana)
Inhale extend RIGHT leg back. Then, exhale bringing the right knee into the nose, engaging the core. Repeat again extending right leg back. 5 rounds recommended. Keep the hips stable throughout as you move with the breath.
Center again and pause in **Downward Dog** Adho Mukha Svanasana
Down Dog Split LEFT LEG Tri Pada Adho Mukha Svanasana (Tri Pada AH-doh MOO-kah-shvah-Nahs-ana)
Inhale extend LEFT leg back. Then, exhale bringing the left knee into the nose, engaging the core. Repeat again extending left leg back. 5 rounds recommended. Keep the hips stable throughout as you move with the breath.

Come to **Hero Pose** Vajrasana (vahj-RAHS-uh-nuh)
Kneeling on the floor, sit on the heels. Inhale arms all the way up. Bring hands down to heart center.

Move into **Gate Pose** RIGHT Parighasana (par-ee-GOSS-anna)
Stretch your right leg out to the right side of the space and press the inside of the foot to the floor. Keep your left knee directly below your left hip so the thigh is perpendicular to the floor.
Revolving Beam Pose RIGHT Parivrtta Parighasana (par-ee-vrt-tah (pahr-eee-GAHS-uh-nuh)
Put your left hand outside of your left ankle with fingers aiming back same as the direction of your toes. With your left palm, press the floor and spread out your fingers.
Raise your rib cage up in the direction of the ceiling. Make an arch by your back to curve your spine. Stretch right arm up over the head; keep extending it back to maintain the curve of the spine. Remain in the position for 30 to 60 seconds and breathe deeply. After that, lower your raised arm and bend your right knee, placing it back next to the left into **Hero Pose** Vajrasana

Switch sides:
Move into **Gate Pose** LEFT Parighasana (par-ee-GOSS-anna)
Stretch your left leg out to the left side of the space and press the inside of the foot to the floor. Keep your right knee directly below your right hip so the thigh is perpendicular to the floor.
Revolving Beam Pose LEFT Parivrtta Parighasana (par-ee-vrt-tah (pahr-eee-GAHS-uh-nuh)
Put your right hand outside of your right ankle with fingers aiming back same as the direction of your toes. With your right palm, press the floor and spread out your fingers. Raise your rib cage up in the direction of the ceiling. Make an arch by your back to curve your spine. Stretch left arm up over the head; keep extending it back to maintain the curve of the spine.

Remain in the position for 30 to 60 seconds and breathe deeply. After that, lower your raised arm and bend your left knee, placing it back next to the right into **Hero Pose** Vajrasana

Stand in **Mountain Pose** Tadasana
Dancing Moon with 2 blocks at the front corners of the mat on their tallest height. Glance to see your blocks are in place for **Half Moon Pose** RIGHT LEG
Ardha Chandrasana (ARD-uh chan-DRAHS-uh-nuh)
Reach through your left hand and then down to the left block. Straighten your left leg while simultaneously lifting your right leg back. Work to bring the right leg parallel to the floor, or even higher than your hips.
Reach actively through your right heel. Take care to not lock the left leg's knee. Stack top hip directly over your bottom hip, and open your torso to the right. Then extend your right arm and point your fingertips directly toward the sky. Balance for a moment. On an exhale, bend the right knee into the torso or core. Extend back again on an inhale. Repeat leg extension 5 times in rhythm with the breath.

Back to **Mountain Pose** Tadasana
Dancing Moon with 2 blocks at the front corners of the mat on their tallest height. Glance to see your blocks are in place for **Half Moon Pose** LEFT LEG
Ardha Chandrasana
Reach through your right hand and then down to the right block. Straighten your right leg while simultaneously lifting your left leg back. Work to bring the left leg parallel to the floor, or even higher than your hips.
Reach actively through your left heel. Take care to not lock the right leg's knee. Stack top hip directly over your bottom hip, and open your torso to the left. Then extend your left arm and point your fingertips directly toward the sky. Balance for a moment. On an exhale, bend the left knee into the torso or core. Extend back again on an inhale. Repeat leg extension 5 times in rhythm with the breath.

Back to **Mountain Pose** Tadasana
Balancing Sequence for strength RIGHT LEG:
With LEFT foot planted firmly into the earth, move into **Tree pose** Vrksasana (vrik-SHAH-suh-nuh) lifting RIGHT Leg, Hands at heart, raise them up and out. Balance.
Warrior I Virabhadrasana I (veer-uh-buh-DRAHS-uh-nuh)
Step the RIGHT foot back about 4 to 5 feet. Turn your left foot out 90 degrees so your toes point to the top of the mat. Pivot your right foot inward at a 45-degree angle. Point your pelvis and torso in the same direction as your right toes are pointing.
Bend your left knee over your left ankle so your shin is perpendicular to the floor. Raise your arms overhead with your palms facing each other.

Warrior III Virabhadrasana III Press your weight into your left foot. Lift your right leg as you lower your torso, bringing your body parallel to the ground. Your arms, still extended, will now reach forward.
Flex the right foot and reach out through your heel.
Straighten your standing leg as you continue to lift the right leg, careful not lock your knee. Stretch your body from your fingertips all the way through your lifted heel. Gaze at the floor a few feet in front of your body.

Transition to **King Dancer Pose** Natarajasana (NOT-ah-rahj-AHS-uh-nuh)
Bring your RIGHT heel toward your right buttock. Reach your right hand down and clasp your right foot's inner ankle. You can also loop a strap around the top of your right foot, and then hold onto the strap with your right hand. Reach your left arm overhead, pointing your fingertips toward the ceiling and facing your palm to the right.
Fix your gaze softly at a **drishti** point or unmoving point of focus. Make sure your left kneecap and toes point directly forward.
When you feel steady, begin to lift your right foot away from your body as you lean your torso slightly forward. Keep your chest lifted and continue reaching your left hand's fingertips up toward the ceiling. Raise your right foot as high as you can.
Come back to **Mountain Pose** Tadasana
Eagle Pose Garudasana (gahr-ooo-DAHS-uh-nuh)
Bend your knees. Balance on your RIGHT foot and cross your left thigh over your right. Fix your gaze at a point in front of you. Hook the top of your left foot behind your right calf. Balance for one breath.
(Omit the foot hook and cross the leg over the top of the standing leg, for a less intense variation)
Extend your arms straight in front of your body. Move your left arm under your right. Bend your elbows, and then raise your forearms perpendicular to the floor. Wrap your hands, and press your palms together (or as close as you can get them). Lift your elbows and reach your fingertips toward the ceiling. Keep your shoulder blades pressing down your back, toward your waist.
Square your hips. Breathe smoothly and evenly.
Hold for up to one minute, focusing on your breath and keeping your gaze fixed and soft. Gently unwind your arms and legs

Back to **Mountain Pose** Tadasana
Balancing Sequence for strength LEFT LEG:
With RIGHT foot planted firmly into the earth, move into **Tree pose** Vrksasana (vrik-SHAH-suh-nuh) lifting LEFT Leg, Hands at heart, raise them up and out. Balance.
Warrior I Virabhadrasana I (veer-uh-buh-DRAHS-uh-nuh)
Step the LEFT foot back about 4 to 5 feet. Turn your right foot out 90 degrees so your toes point to the top of the mat. Pivot your left foot inward at a 45-degree angle. Point your pelvis and torso in the same direction as your left toes are pointing.
Bend your right knee over your right ankle so your shin is perpendicular to the floor. Raise your arms overhead with your palms facing each other.

Warrior III Virabhadrasana III Press your weight into your right foot. Lift your left leg as you lower your torso, bringing your body parallel to the ground. Your arms, still extended, will now reach forward.
Flex the left foot and reach out through your heel.
Straighten your standing leg as you continue to lift the left leg, careful not lock your knee. Stretch your body from your fingertips all the way through your lifted heel. Gaze at the floor a few feet in front of your body.

Transition to **King Dancer Pose** Natarajasana (NOT-ah-rahj-AHS-uh-nuh)
Bring your LEFT heel toward your left buttock. Reach your left hand down and clasp your left foot's inner ankle. You can also loop a strap around the top of your left foot, and then hold onto the strap with your left hand. Reach your right arm overhead, pointing your fingertips toward the ceiling and facing your palm to the left.
Fix your gaze softly at a **drishti** point or unmoving point of focus. Make sure your right kneecap and toes point directly forward.
When you feel steady, begin to lift your left foot away from your body as you lean your torso slightly forward. Keep your chest lifted and continue reaching your right hand's fingertips up toward the ceiling. Raise your left foot as high as you can.
Come back to **Mountain Pose** Tadasana
Eagle Pose Garudasana (gahr-ooo-DAHS-uh-nuh)
Bend your knees. Balance on your LEFT foot and cross your right thigh over your left. Fix your gaze at a point in front of you. Hook the top of your right foot behind your left calf. Balance for one breath.
(Omit the foot hook and cross the leg over the top of the standing leg, for a less intense variation)
Extend your arms straight in front of your body. Move your right arm under your left. Bend your elbows, and then raise your forearms perpendicular to the floor. Wrap your hands, and press your palms together (or as close as you can get them). Lift your elbows and reach your fingertips toward the ceiling. Keep your shoulder blades pressing down your back, toward your waist.
Square your hips. Breathe smoothly and evenly.
Hold for up to one minute, focusing on your breath and keeping your gaze fixed and soft. Gently unwind your arms and legs

Stand in **Mountain Pose** Tadasana
Crow Pose Bakasana (bah-KAHS-uh-nuh)
Bring your palms to the mat, shoulder-distance apart. Spread your fingers and press evenly across both palms. Press your shins against the back of your upper arms. Draw your knees in as close to your underarms as possible.
Lift onto the balls of your feet as you lean forward. Round your back and draw your core in firmly. Look at the floor between your hands or at a point even more forward, if possible. *You can use a block between your hands and place your head on the block for balance.
As you continue to lean forward, lift your feet off the floor and draw your heels toward your buttocks. Try lifting one foot and then the other. Balance your

torso and legs on the back of your upper arms. Touch your big toes together. Draw your belly in. Breathe steadily.
Advanced: Begin to straighten your elbows. Keep your knees and shins hugging in tightly toward your armpits. Keep your forearms drawn firmly toward the midline of your body.

Half Frog Pose RIGHT & LEFT Ardha Bhekasana (ARD-uh Beh-KAHS-an-nuh)
Bend your right knee and bring the heel toward the same-side buttock. Then, supporting yourself on the left forearm, reach back with your right hand and clasp the inside of your foot. As you slowly rotate your elbow toward the ceiling, slide your fingers over the top of the foot and curl them over the toe tips. The base of your palm should be pressing the top of the foot.
Square your shoulders with the front of the mat and don't collapse into your left shoulder. Instead, press down with your elbow to lift your chest.
Change side: Bend your left knee and bring the heel toward the same-side buttock. Then, supporting yourself on the right forearm, reach back with your left hand and clasp the inside of your foot. As you slowly rotate your elbow toward the ceiling, slide your fingers over the top of the foot and curl them over the toe tips. The base of your palm should be pressing the top of the foot.
Square your shoulders with the front of the mat and don't collapse into your right shoulder. Instead, press down with your elbow to lift your chest.

Release the entire body down for **Relaxation Pose** Savasana (sha-VAHS-ah-nuh)
Allow legs to fall naturally to the sides. Eyes closed and relaxed.
Give yourself time to just be.

Closing Meditation
true self

In this meditation we will connect to our own true self, with our inner selves.
We will work to strengthen this connection. Your true self is always with you and it takes practice to tune into it.
As you strengthen this connection, you will be guided towards better choices in life and to live your life as your very best self.

Bring your attention to your breath. Allow the abdomen to expand as you inhale.
Exhale slowly, allowing your body to relax on the exhale.
As you breathe, create a stillness in your mind.
If you have any unwanted thoughts during this meditation, just say in your mind, "Not now."
Close your eyes and visualize yourself sitting on a cloud. Imagine a network of small clouds around you, all connected to the light that lives inside you.

Imagine your true self as a powerful glowing angel above you; this is who you really are. As you observe this angel, it smiles and glows with light.
Ask this angel, your true self, to unite with you now.
Feel yourself uniting with your true self at your crown chakra, the very top of your head.
Feel it as a download into your consciousness.
Is there anything your true self is telling you?
Is there a question you have for your true self?

Allow your mind to be still to receive any feelings or responses, images, or ideas. Perhaps you feel just a knowing or a sense of comfort. Let these feelings or messages develop and filter into your mind.

You now have made a very special and profound connection.
As you practice this meditation, it will become easier for you to connect with your true self and receive daily guidance when you need it.
Each day, clear your mind, set an intention and connect with your true self whenever you need some strength.

Move Chill Yoga
Portable Yoga Class Plan 12
strength & balance

Diamond Pose
Table Pose
Dancing Cat Right & Left
Revolving Planks Right & Left
Downward Dog
Dancing Dog Right & Left
Hero Pose
Gate Pose RIGHT
Revolving Beam Pose RIGHT
Hero Pose
Gate Pose LEFT
Revolving Beam Pose LEFT
Hero Pose
Mountain Pose
Dancing Moon RIGHT
Mountain
Dancing Moon LEFT
Mountain

Balancing Sequence: Right leg	Balancing Sequence: Left leg
Tree Pose	Tree Pose
Warrior I	Warrior I
Warrior III	Warrior III
King Dancer Pose	King Dancer Pose
Mountain Pose	Mountain Pose
Eagle Pose	Eagle Pose
Mountain Pose	Mountain Pose

Crow Pose
Half Frog Pose Right & Left
Relaxation Pose

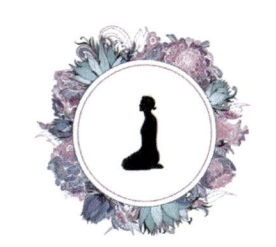

playlists ☾ ✴ ☀

1
Concentrate on Calm	Deep Sleep Walkers
Kusanagi	ODESZA
In a Forest with leaves in your hair	Sad Souls
Fade Into You (Instrumental)	Korey Dane
Cloud Speed	Sad Souls
For What It's Worth	DJ Drez
The Dream of the Dolphin	Enigma
Ong Namo – I Bow	Gurunam Singh
Million Reasons (Instrumental)	Adriana Vitale
Nightvision	Daft Punk
Infinite Cosmos	Meditation Music

2
I feel It Coming (Instrumental)	KPH
Holograms	M83
Begin Again	The Piano Guys
Chandelier (Instrumental)	Steve Petrunak
With or Without You	Regency Philharmonic Orchestra
Memory of Trees	Enya
You are All I See	Active Child
The Sun Shines Only for Me	Fairmont
Stella Blue (Instrumental)	Bradford Hoopes
Sign of the Times (Instrumental)	KPH
Snow Dress	Sad Souls

3
Moonlit Images	Massage Tribe
Touch The Sky (Instrumentsl)	Daniel Jang
Claire de Lune	Claude Debussy
Forever Young (Instrumental)	The Professionals
Dagkar Taso Mila's Cave	Tibetan Meditation Music
To Build a Home	The Cinematic Orchestra
Wild Horses	The Sundays
Badagary Beach	Ben Onono
Saturn	Sleeping at Last
Stay With Me (Instrumental)	The Highend Karaoke
Frog from Interloper	Carbon Based Life Forms

4
Fluffy Clouds	Joe Fish
Morning Dew	Grateful Dead
First Day of My Life	Bright Eyes
Burgs	Mt. Wolf
Bailero	Sarah Brightman
Shriman Narayan (Instrumental)	Kishore Kumar & Dr. Ramachandra Murthy
Big Sur	Porcelain Raft
Catch & Release	Matt Simons
Happy	Bruce Springsteen
There Will Be Time	Mumford & Sons & Baaba Maal
Horizon of Gold	Ben Leinbachl & Jai Uttal
"I"	Ben Jordan

NOTES

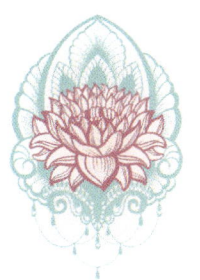

Printed in Great Britain
by Amazon